Fat to Fit Without Dieting

Jeanne Rhodes

CB

CONTEMPORARY
BOOKS

CHICAGO

Library of Congress Cataloging-in-Publication Data

Rhodes, Jeanne,
    Fat to fit without dieting : the no-diet eating plan that burns
off excess fat forever / Jeanne Rhodes.
      p.   cm.
    ISBN 0-8092-4158-7
    1. Reducing.   I. Title.
RM222.2R467   1990
613.2′5—dc20   90-35875
                                          CIP

Published by Contemporary Books, Inc.
180 North Michigan Avenue, Chicago, Illinois 60601
Manufactured in the United States of America
International Standard Book Number: 0-8092-4158-7

In one week you could be losing weight and experiencing an unbelievable increase in energy! Whether you have 100 pounds or 10 pounds to lose, the simple but scientific concepts presented in *Fat To Fit Without Dieting* will show you how to decrease body fat stores and body fat production *permanently*. In following the program you will eat foods you enjoy, lose weight comfortably and increase your energy level without the discomfort and health risks of dieting.

No food is eliminated as you learn to work in harmony with your body's weight-regulating mechanism to lose body fat and weight comfortably, and never go hungry or be overweight again!

Following are some of the highlights:

- You must not go hungry!

- No calorie counting, no weighing and measuring of foods, no elimination of favorite foods.

- Delicious meals and snacks planned for you, or if you prefer, detailed guidelines for planning your own.

- Eat your favorite foods in a scientifically proven way that will increase calorie burning and reduce body fat.

- Your "Binge" day – have a banana split or lobster with melted butter!

- Special "Quick Weight Loss" plan for those in a hurry.

- "Overindulgences" happen to everyone on occasion – fat or thin! Learn about the special remedy that will prevent yours from causing a weight gain!

- Scientifically designed methods to increase metabolism and fat burning for as long as 15-20 hours!

ACKNOWLEDGMENTS

I gratefully acknowledge all the wonderful people who have gone through the "Fat to Fit Without Dieting" program allowing me to share in the transformation, not only of their bodies and their health but of their lives as well. I relive the joy of success with my own weight problems through each and every one, and to them I will always be grateful for their contribution to my own personal growth.

I'm especially indebted to Cynthia Hart, who has played a significant role in the success of the Jeanne Rhodes Wellness Center. In assisting her to end her weight problems, I have experienced one of those very special friendships that you hold in your heart and cherish in your life.

A special acknowledgment goes to my husband, John, who inspired and encouraged the writing of this book. His unconditional love helped renew and revitalize me when I felt frustrated, overwhelmed, and very unlovable. Knowing he was there when I needed him was a wonderful refuge and comfort throughout the many months of writing, rewriting, and total absorption in this manuscript. To him, I would like to say a very special "Thank You."

TABLE OF CONTENTS

1

MY LIFETIME PROBLEM WITH FAT

I weighed 185 pounds when I attempted, for what seemed like the 50th time, to lose weight again. But this time was different in many ways. There was no dieting – I wasn't counting calories, eating special foods or going hungry and even my energy level was beginning to increase.

I was eating all my favorite foods so I did not experience the usual *rush* to lose weight so that I could get back to eating "regular" food again. Always before, I hadn't worried about *keeping* the weight off, just *getting* it off, and the faster the better!

I always fell for the promise of "fast" weight loss, without realizing that I was already an expert at fast weight loss, having done it many times over! This time the pounds came off a little slower but the weight loss was steady, and to my delight, I reached my goal of 125 pounds in less than a year. But more importantly, for the first time in my life, I was successful in keeping the weight off and at present I have maintained my desired weight for ten years – all without dieting!

This accomplishment still seems miraculous to me, having spent over 30 years of my life fighting the scales, losing weight over and over again with each new diet which always failed, leaving me

5-10 pounds heavier than I was before. There were many seemingly dead-end questions that were confusing and totally frustrating. If I lost weight the first week or two on a diet, why did I stop losing after the next few weeks on *exactly* the same food intake? And why did I very quickly gain back the lost weight plus a few pounds extra after each diet attempt?

These and many more were the perplexing, unanswerable questions that were part of each dieting failure and I had to find some answers. In desperation, I turned to research and intensive study in an attempt to find a solution to my weight problem. It took years of formal education, plus patience and perseverance to find the answers I needed. But little by little, I found the research and information that enabled me to finally win my 30 year battle with fat.

After my own success came a great desire to use the new, exciting research information I had found to design a weight control program to help other people who were having the same problems I once had. It was my dream to inspire and help as many people as I could who had experienced frustrations and failures with weight control, and today that dream has come true. There are hundreds of men, women and children who have been successful in losing weight and maintaining their weight goals by following the "Fat To Fit Without Dieting" program, which forms the basis of this book. I sincerely believe that part of this tremendous success is due to my personal experience with the very real problem of being severely overweight.

My own problems with weight began early in my childhood and I will share some of these experiences with you, most of which you will probably identify with very quickly.

A Fat Childhood

Having lived most of my life as a fat person, I know first hand what it's like. Even as a five-year old, I was fat. Not chubby – just plain fat. I was one of those fat children who had never been thin, and by the time I was nine, even my mother was desperate, and sought the help of my pediatrician. He decided that I was entirely too heavy and introduced me to my first low calorie diet. I had never been a big eater, and much to my surprise, the low calorie diet he put me on allowed more food than I was already eating! Needless to say, I didn't lose any weight. It was at this point that he felt there might be a glandular problem. After the appropriate tests, he determined that I had a low metabolic rate due perhaps to a sluggish thyroid. He instructed my mother to continue my diet, and added thyroid medication, a combination which he felt most assuredly, would produce a loss of weight. Although only nine, I felt elated that the doctor had seemingly found a reason for my weight problem and hopefully, with the thyroid medication, I could look forward to being like other children. I didn't like the restrictions that being fat placed on me. I wanted to wear attractive clothes like the other children wore, and I wanted to run as fast and climb as easily as the others. I had many friends and they seemed to pay little attention to my weight, but I felt uneasy being so different than they. I was the only fat child around, and to make matters worse, both of my brothers were very thin and neither of my parents were heavy.

Being fat not only disturbed me, but I found out much to my dismay, that it was also very much a concern to both of my parents. My mother had to buy women's dresses for me and attempt to alter the waist and skirt lengths to fit a nine year old. There were no "chubby" sized clothes for fat children in our small town. On one occasion, my mother was attempting to alter a woman's size 18 dress for me to wear to a special school event. The shoulders were too wide, the waist was too long, and the skirt was almost to the floor. In sheer desperation, she made a statement I'll never forget, "If you weren't so fat, I could dress you in cute clothes like the other little girls wear!" I was shocked and hurt as I realized then that my being fat was bothering her almost as much as it was bothering me. To make matters worse, the thyroid medication did not help my weight problem, and had to be discontinued when I began to show an intolerance to it, which probably meant I hadn't needed it in the first place.

At eleven years of age, I weighed in at a whopping 165 pounds! I began trying one diet after another and by the time I had reached my teens, I had tried every diet I could get my hands on. Nothing worked. Since all the diets had failed, I knew of only one way left to lose weight. I would stop eating. That *had* to work! There was no way to fail if you didn't eat! And so I began living primarily on toast and tea with very little else. I became anemic, but I lost the weight and that was all I could think about. I was thin for the first time in my life! I could wear attractive clothes, I became a majorette in the high school band, I got the lead part in the senior play, and I was even on the girl's varsity basketball and softball teams. I was on a high – plenty of dates, popular, and loving every minute of it! A boy in my high school senior class, who had been a classmate since my earlier "fat days," told me that I reminded him of the Ugly Duckling that had turned into a beautiful swan.

Ironically, my parents were now desperately trying to get me to eat, taking me to our family doctor on several occasions, enlisting his aid in trying to convince me that I was ruining my health. One such occasion I can remember as if it were only yesterday. Sitting patiently in the doctor's office, as he attempted to explain the life-threatening dangers of my starvation approach to losing weight, I waited until he paused for a response from me. I could see both shock and resignation on his face when I told him matter-of-factly, "I appreciate the time you've spent with me, but I've tried your low calorie diets and they don't work. This is the only thing that has worked for me, and I would rather die than be fat again." At the time, I meant just that. As a young teenager the possibility of death or illness held little or no meaning for me, but being fat did. All I knew was that for the first time in my life, I was like the other "normal" teenagers. Being like your peers and being attractive are both very strong drives in the teen years, and I was no exception. How ironic that not too many years before, I had been sitting in a pediatrician's office as he accused me of "sneaking" food, eating too much, and insisting that nothing but overeating was causing my weight problem! There was no way I could convince him that I was not eating too much or "sneaking" food. Dieting had produced no weight loss, just a lot of deprivation, hunger and false accusations. I was determined that I would never be falsely accused in that manner again. But the future was not as bright as I had thought.

Anorexia!

After high school, part of the motivation that prompted me to go into Nurses Training was the search for a healthier way to control my weight. Unfortunately, the nutrition education was little more than that offered in most high school Home Economics classes, and included nothing about nutrition that was of help to me.

I continued my dietary routine of toast and tea with bits of other food on occasion for several years. Every time I tried adding more food to my diet, I would gain 5-10 pounds very quickly, after which I would return to my old stand-by of toast and tea again. Finally, in my 20's, I was admitted to Johns Hopkins Hospital, anorexic and with a life-threatening illness. The doctor delivered his message in a very blunt manner – "Either you start eating or you will die." The reality of his statement finally dawned on me and I knew I would have to make some changes. By this time, I had two young children and much to live for.

Fat Again

I began eating a very carefully controlled low calorie diet. But once again the weight began increasing and continued to increase until I was overweight again. I tried every new fad diet I could find in a futile attempt to control the weight, but failed with each dieting attempt. Over and over again, I would lose weight only to regain what I had lost, and then some, until I finally reached 185 pounds!

Finding The Answer

In desperation I turned to the study of nutrition. I had to find some answers. And find some answers, I did! Some very exciting answers that make losing weight relatively easy – much easier than I ever expected. This book will explain those things and the Eating Plan step by step so that anyone can lose weight without counting calories, without going hungry, and without eliminating any favorite foods, just as the many people in the "Fat To Fit" program have done.

A Happy Ending

As I write these words, I am fifty-three years old, going on thirty nine! My cholesterol count is 131, my blood pressure is 110/68, and my weight has remained stable at 125 pounds for ten years. I enjoy an extremely busy schedule presenting Nutrition Seminars throughout the East Coast, instructing ten one-hour aerobic classes, four "Fat To Fit" classes weekly and co-owning, with my husband John, Gold's Professional Health and Fitness Center.

My life has been very rewarding. I am constantly re-living my success in the battle against obesity as I see the joy in people I work with, who are succeeding in transforming themselves into healthier, slimmer, attractive, and more importantly – happier people.

Questions
My Lifetime Problem With Fat

You lost 60 pounds. How long did it take you to lose this much?

It was less than a year, but exactly how many months, I cannot say with accuracy. I was so absorbed in researching, studying and using myself as a "guinea pig" to test the information, that I did not keep track of the exact time it took for me to lose the weight.

How did the "Fat to Fit Without Dieting" program come into being?

I had spent quite a few years in search and study and finally found limited but valid information and research on the effects of dieting. Using the information, I began a weight loss program, and continued to study. From each new bit of information and research I learned a little more to make losing weight more effective and even a little easier. There were times, however, that I would run into "snags" and the weight loss would stop, or I would even gain. Immediately I would begin searching again for additional information and research to find out why. Having learned quite a lot by the time the weight was lost, I was anxious to continue my study as it applied to other people. The next several years were spent studying and compiling additional research data and information, part of which resulted from my work with other overweight people who, like me, had their own unique problems. As a result, a new "no diet" approach to weight control evolved and was proving successful for every participant following the plan. These outstanding results prompted the next step which was to put the tried and proven effective plan into a complete program that overweight persons could utilize comfortably to become permanently trim. The program was developed and appropriately named "Fat To Fit Without Dieting" and has been extremely successful. As a sequel this book was written allowing even more people to achieve a permanent metabolic improvement to bring about normal weight and allow normal eating.

Had you lost weight before?

Yes! Many times! Unfortunately I always gained it back *with interest*. There were times when I kept the weight off for as long as a year and a half while, through sheer willpower, living on a particular fad diet. I kept the weight off even longer when I became anorexic, but it almost cost me my life.

The worst part of dieting was the feeling that after all the struggle and deprivation to lose, I never felt in control. The lack of permanence – never knowing when the diet would stop working and when it did, as they all do, not knowing how to prevent all the weight from coming back on. As an overweight person I felt very much "out of control."

Have you had any weight fluctuations since your weight "normalized" ten years ago?

On occasion, I have gained three or four pounds, but the nice part is that now I know exactly why, and I know exactly what to do to get it back off. If I gain, it's usually during a vacation or extended holidays. I will not allow myself more than a four-pound gain simply because I do not feel as energetic or as comfortable in my clothes.

What do you feel is your most important psychological benefit from your ten years at a normal weight?

There are many, many, psychological benefits, but for me one of the most important is the feeling of being in control of my life. Knowing and understanding certain of the physiological and bio-chemical principles of the body has put me in control of my weight which has given me a certain feeling of control in most other aspects of my life. There may be some overweight people who do not feel the same, but the people I've worked with will invariably identify with this "out of control" feeling. The sad truth is an overweight body usually projects this same message to others and many times has a negative effect on credibility as well as capability.

For what reason did you wait ten years after losing weight to write a book?

Several reasons. I needed to find research information to validate some of the things I had experienced. As a professional, information must be substantiated by proven research information, not just personal experience and opinion.

I also felt that losing the excess weight was only the first phase, and that maintaining that weight loss for a minimum of five years was essential in helping prove the method as effective. Many people lose weight, but it cannot be considered "permanent" unless their weight remains normal for a period of approximately five years.

Also, I needed time to work with other people in weight loss situations to discover, study and address other problem areas that had not been part of my weight loss experience.

Why do you feel you spent almost 40 years as a fat person before you found an answer to your weight problem?

Forty years ago, or even thirty years ago, overweight problems were not as prevalent as they are today. When I was an overweight child, I was the only one in my neighborhood, and it was unusual at that time to see an overweight child anywhere. Today, there are many overweight children and their numbers as well as the number of obese adults are increasing rapidly.

With larger numbers of overweight people, use of a dieting approach for weight control was evaluated and found to produce an alarming failure rate of 99.5%. This prompted researchers to begin investigating, and it was found that this method of weight control was useless. Today, even the media – magazines, newspapers, television, etc. – are reporting research results that consistently find dieting ineffective for weight control.

My search began over twenty years ago when obesity was not as prevalent. Diets were being recommended for weight control and failure was viewed as a lack of willpower on the part of the dieter! Much of today's research on dieting had not yet been done, and most of today's concepts were unknown. It was tedious and time consuming for me to find even small bits of information that could be used to shed some light on the problem. The study of physiological and biochemical functions of the body formed a basis but other information which is readily available today, was very difficult to find and usually incomplete, so that a "piecing together" from several sources was necessary.

On several occasions I experienced particular physiological occurrences and then had to wait two or three years for research to validate my observations.

Counting the years of formal education plus the years of study and research of my own, *Fat To Fit Without Dieting* is a culmination of a total of more than 20 years of study.

2

METABOLISM: THE KEY TO WEIGHT CONTROL

Metabolism refers to all the biochemical processes involved in breaking down the food you eat for bodily functions and energy.

The rate of speed and efficiency of your metabolism is called the metabolic rate. In simple terms, metabolic rate is the rate at which your body burns calories for energy.

No two bodies are exactly alike, nor do they function quite the same. Metabolic rates have a natural variance from one person to another – some are faster, some are slower and others are at different degrees in between.

How Your Metabolism Works

To understand how your metabolism works, we might compare it with the thermostat on your furnace. If you turn the thermostat up, it uses more fuel, turn it down and it uses less fuel. Your body's fuel is the calorie. A fast metabolism may be thought of as being set on "high" and uses more calories (fuel), while a slow metabolism, set on low, uses fewer calories. Calories that are not used for

11

energy are stored as fat. If you have a slow metabolism, you use fewer calories for energy which means more will be stored as fat. A fast metabolism uses more calories for energy and little is left over to be stored as fat.

If you are overweight, chances are you have a slow metabolism which means you are using fewer calories for energy and leaving more to be stored as body fat.

Thin People Eat More Calories!!

When I make the statement at a "Fat to Fit" seminar, that thin people eat more than overweight people I can see the puzzled looks on the faces of the audience. Then I ask how many of them know a thin person who eats twice as much or more than they do. Hands go up all over the auditorium as the puzzled looks on their faces turn into knowing grins.

Based on the latest research findings, most thin people eat an estimated average of 600 calories *more* per day than overweight people. The thin person's metabolism burns calories at a faster rate, leaving fewer to be stored as fat. On the other hand, the fat individual may eat fewer calories, but having a slower metabolism, will burn the calories slowly and more are left to be stored as fat.

For this reason, an excess of body fat must be viewed as a *symptom* of a slower than normal metabolism. Dieting is an attempt to treat only the symptom, and treating symptoms is a no-win situation. For example, if you had appendicitis, one of the *symptoms* would be pain. Your doctor could treat this symptom with pain killing medication, but in the meantime, the cause of the pain, the appendicitis, will only get worse. The only solution is to treat the cause, which is the appendicitis, and the pain-related symptom will abate permanently.

Excess body fat is a *symptom*, which is caused by a slower than normal metabolism. You cannot treat the symptom, you must treat the *cause*. The slow metabolism must be increased so that calories will be burned faster, and less body fat will be produced. Correcting the *cause* will result in permanent normalization of weight. This is the only way; anything else is "putting a band-aid on the sore" and at best will be only temporary.

If you have a weight problem, dieting will aggravate the problem, or may actually have created the problem in the first place. Cutting back to low calorie fare will alter your metabolism. Even if you have a *normal* metabolism, dieting will slow it down making weight control more difficult than it was before dieting. If you have a *slow* metabolism to begin with, each dieting attempt will slow it down even more. Eventually you will reach the point where you will never be able to eat like a normal person again. In fact, in some research studies, people with a history of repetitive dieting have reached the point where they do not lose weight, even on an 800 calorie-per-day diet! Ironically their problem was created by the dieting itself. Dieting will sabotage your weight control efforts in many ways and I will explain these more fully in the next chapter.

Slowing A Normal Metabolism

There may be many of you who never had a weight problem until recently. Evidently you didn't have a slow metabolism, so why do you have a weight problem now? Is it possible that your previously normal metabolism has changed?

Yes, it most definitely is possible to slow down a normal metabolism which will in turn create problems with weight control. Consider the following dieting disaster:

A 32 year old woman is five feet five inches tall, weighs 125 pounds and has never had a weight problem. Unknowingly, she begins making certain lifestyle changes which precipitate an increase in her previously stable body weight. Because of her very busy schedule she soon begins skipping breakfast and occasionally even lunch. At the end of the day she is ravenous and an overabundance of food is consumed at the evening meal which, to save time, often includes "convenience" foods most of which are usually very high in fat. Along with the development of these fat producing eating habits there is also a decrease in exercise – she feels she no longer can spare the time. As a result, her weight slowly begins to increase. By the age of 33, this woman notices she has gained 12 pounds over the past year. It is Spring and bathing suit weather is fast approaching. Wanting to lose those 12 pounds quickly, she cuts her calorie intake to 900 a day. Within four weeks, she's lost the weight, but she's paid a price! Of the 12 pounds she lost, only 6 pounds was fat. She also lost 3 pounds of lean tissue and 3 pounds of water. When Fall arrives and the revealing bathing suit is put away, she gradually resumes her old eating habits, becomes less active and the 12 pounds are quickly regained. Little does she realize that she has taken the first step in becoming chronically overweight! The 12 pounds regained are 2/3 fat – 8 pounds of fat plus 4 pounds of water. Her body fat has been increased and her metabolism has been decreased through the dieting itself. With the slight metabolic decrease, by the time Spring arrives the next year, she has an additional 3 pounds added to the original 12 pounds, making a total of 15 pounds of excess weight. She finds that to lose the weight she must cut calories even more drastically than before. Dieting away these 15 pounds, she loses 7 pounds of fat, 4 pounds of lean tissue and 4 pounds of water, which she subsequently regains as 14 pounds of fat and 4 pounds of water, with a futher decrease in metabolic rate ending up at *18* pounds overweight. By this time, she's well on her way to a serious weight problem and ironic as it may seem, each dieting attempt will continue to intensify her problem.

Each time she loses weight through dieting, she will: 1) subsequently regain a little more than she lost; 2) increase her body fat; and 3) slow down her metabolism. Consequently, by her early forties, she will have a serious weight problem, and remembering her younger "thin days," will blame her weight problems on age.

There are four things occurring in the above situation, either one of which will compound weight problems, and with all four at work simultaneously, the results are disastrous! First, there is a naturally occurring 1/2 percent slow down, per year, in metabolism from approximately age 26 on. Second, a metabolic reduction always accompanies a drastic cut in calories. Third, there is approximately a 5 percent increase in weight following each diet attempt. In fact, studies of not only the obese, but also of normal-weight people who followed low calorie diets for only a few weeks show as much as a 15 to 30 percent reduction in metabolism. Fourth, when weight is lost through dieting, part of that weight is lean tissue, but when regained, is mostly fat. Therefore, the dieting itself has increased fat and decreased lean tissue.

Lean Tissue - A "Calorie Burner"

Compounding the weight problems produced by a drop in metabolism is the loss of lean tissue. Lean tissue uses extra calories and losing lean tissue through dieting means that fewer calories will be needed. This is one of the primary reasons men not only require more calories to maintain weight but will usually lose weight faster than women. By nature, men have a much higher percentage of lean tissue than women which increases their calorie requirements. The same is true for women with firm bodies. A decrease in body fat and an increase in lean tissue is necessary for a firm body and will also increase the number of calories needed.

When weight is lost through dieting, the end result is a weight regain and while lean tissue was lost it is fat that is regained. Paradoxically, dieting produces exactly the opposite of what you want – you lose the compact calorie burning muscle and gain fat, ("flab") which takes up more space and uses practically no calories!

One pound of fat takes up approximately *five times* the space of one pound of lean muscle! You may see two people of the same height and weight, and yet one appears "chubby" and the other doesn't. The larger one has more body fat which weighs less than lean but takes more space. It is much like comparing feathers and stones. While one pound of feathers *weighs* the same as one pound of stones, the pound of feathers takes up more space. A perfect example of this is a young friend of mine who weighs 136 pounds at 5 feet 4 inches in height – slightly above the recommended ideal weight for a 5 foot 4 inch female. Yet, her tight firm body has little fat and her measurements, 34-22-34, are indeed ideal! Keep this in mind as you lose weight. Aim for a particular size and a firm, tight body, rather than a particular weight!

Increasing Metabolism

Now I want to address a question that is probably uppermost on your mind concerning your own weight problem:

Can an overweight person increase a slow metabolism, eat like a normal person without dieting, and still lose weight?

The answer to this question is an emphatic *"Yes!"* Anyone

following the program as directed in this book will increase metabolism to burn calories for energy rather than store them as fat. You will enjoy pleasurable eating without dieting while losing weight and keeping it off forever. You will lose *only* fat which results in weight loss *plus* an even more dramatic loss of inches. Your lean muscle tissue will increase slightly to give you a firm body which will not only look better but will burn more calories, and at a faster rate. This means you may require more calories to maintain your desired weight than you ever did as a fat person. I've seen it happen to hundreds of people just as it happened to me, and I was a fat person for over 30 years!

Questions
Metabolism - The Key To Weight Control

My sister is very thin and I am 30 pounds overweight, yet she eats almost twice as much as I do! How can this be?

Your metabolism, or rate at which you burn calories, is much lower than hers. This means you will use fewer calories than she does for all your body processes, so that you will store more as fat. For example, imagine two campfires. One is just barely smoldering with one or two partial pieces of charred logs still glowing. The second is brightly burning and crackling sounds can be heard as the flames reach high around three large, dry logs. Now, imagine you put a handful of twigs on the smoldering one and an equal handful of twigs on the second brightly burning one. Which would "burn up" the twigs faster? Naturally the first campfire which is burning very slowly (slow metabolism) will burn the twigs (calories) much slower, while the brightly burning one (fast metabolism) will burn that handful of twigs very quickly plus much more.

The solution to a weight problem must include some means to increase metabolism. Weight loss by any other method will not only be temporary, but will aggravate and intensify the problem itself.

What causes a slow metabolism?

In many cases, a slow metabolism is part of a normal person's genetic inheritance. Just as some people are born with blue eyes, and some with brown, so it is that some people are born with a fast metabolism and some with a slow metabolism. This does not mean that a slow metabolism is "unhealthy," but just slower by nature than some others. When coping with the many famines and food shortages in years past, the slower metabolism was very fuel efficient – a definite asset for survival. However, in most of today's world, overweight is more of a health hazard than food shortage and a slow metabolism is no longer an asset.

Another cause of a slow metabolism is a naturally occurring slow-down of 1/2 percent, per year from approximately age 26 on. As a result, people in their late 20's, without prior weight problems, may begin very slowly to increase body fat. For the first few years the 1/2 percent metabolic slow-down each year, produces an increase in body fat that is so small it may not be noticed. But, by the mid or late thirties this small yearly slow-down begins to add up, with weight increases and accumulations of body fat becoming obvious in all the wrong places. An attempt to correct the problem through dieting slows the metabolism even more and in many cases creates a weight problem where none existed before.

Regardless of origin, any weight problem will be intensified by dieting and can be corrected – but only by working with the body to increase the metabolism.

If my metabolism is already slow, what effect will dieting have?

If you have a slow metabolism to begin with, each time you go on a diet, you will slow it down even more. Eventually, you may reach the point where you will never be able to eat like a normal person again.

One lady I know who went to a weight control clinic at a leading university did not lose weight even though she was permitted only several servings of rice a day. She was finally given an even more rigid starvation diet of 1/2 grapefruit 3 times daily before she began losing weight. The weight she lost was quickly regained, plus more, after she had returned home. She had spent thousands of dollars to end up with her metabolism even slower, and an increase in weight! At this writing she is in the "Fat To Fit" program, has lost over 56 pounds, is still averaging a loss of 1-2 pounds weekly, has had her insulin medication cut in half, and her blood pressure medication totally eliminated. She is eating more than she did before losing weight and none of her favorite foods have been eliminated.

Why did my doctor put me on a low calorie diet to lose weight?

Doctors receive very little or no nutrition education. I can remember as a nurse it was very embarrassing to be asked a question about nutrition. I had received very little education in that field, and yet most people expected me, as a nurse, to know about nutrition.

With all the new research on drugs, diseases, medical procedures, treatments, etc., it is almost impossible for medical doctors to keep abreast of all the new material and research just in medicine alone. For this reason, it seems unreasonable to expect them to be just as expert in nutrition.

In her book, *Let's Get Well,* Adelle Davis, a consulting nutritionist, wrote about doctor-prescribed diets. She said the American Medical Association and the American Dietetic Association have both pointed out that because of a lack of nutrition education, doctors usually copy diets from text books which reflect more tradition than scientific fact, and are not based on current research findings.

I seem to gain a little more with each diet I try. Why do I regain more weight after I go off a diet, and end up heavier than I was before I started?

Dieting slows down your metabolism a little more with each subsequent diet. In fact, in a recent research study, even *normal-weight* people who dieted for only a few weeks had a 15-30 percent reduction in metabolism. This means you are burning calories at an even slower rate than you did before the diet. When you begin eating the same calories as before, you will be burning them slower, and more will be used for fat storage and less for energy, which will cause an increase in body fat and weight.

In addition, fat producing enzymes, AT-LPL for example, will be four or more times more active in their fat storing activities after dieting than before, which will also add to weight increases.

To top it all off, lean tissue is part of the weight lost through dieting. Lean tissue is a "calorie burner," requiring many more calories than fat tissue. Fat tissue increases, replacing the lost lean tissue when weight is regained after a diet.

Studies show that there is an average increase of 5% in total weight after a diet attempt, so you are very typical in gaining back more than you lost after dieting. This is part of the futility and frustration of dieting.

You say that too much body fat must be viewed as a symptom of a slower than normal metabolism. Is this always true? I have an overweight friend who eats a lot of food!

I have a very thin brother who eats a tremendous amount of food! I also work with people on weight gain programs and many times it is harder for these people to gain weight than it is for others to lose weight. Their metabolic rates seem to automatically increase when their food intake increases dramatically, as if "programmed" to maintain a certain body weight. This kind of metabolic function does not occur in the overweight person who usually gains weight very easily.

I am not suggesting that your friend can constantly overindulge and still lose weight. While it is possible to increase to normal, it is not possible to change a slow metabolism to a fast metabolism. It will probably never function exactly like the thin person's, but with proper eating and activity it will increase to a rate that is within a normal range, allowing a normal weight to be reached and maintained comfortably.

Is it easier for an overweight person who has never dieted to lose weight than it is for the person who had dieted and regained weight several times?

Yes. Overweight people who have never dieted before are rare, but in my experience in working with these people, weight loss occurs a little easier and is more consistent on a week to week basis. The frequent dieter can increase metabolism, but must be a little more diligent in following the program and weekly weight loss is not as consistent, because the metabolism is usually much slower. Also, body fat percentage is higher since each dieting failure produces a decrease in lean tissue and a subsequent increase in fat tissue. All of these things tend to make metabolic increases a little more difficult, but certainly not impossible for the person who has been a frequent dieter.

Why is it so important to lose weight slowly?

Losing weight slowly, and inches more dramatically, usually is a good indicator that metabolism is increasing and fat, not lean tissue, is being lost, which is your goal in making weight loss *permanent*. The average body can only metabolize approximately 1-2 pounds of fat a week. A greater loss than that usually suggests that lean tissue (which is heavier) is accountable for part of the lost weight. Loss of lean tissue will lower caloric requirement, which in turn may stop weight loss.

One pound of fat takes up five times the space of one pound of lean. They both weigh one pound but the fat occupies five times the space – much like comparing feathers and stones. It is for this reason that inches lost are very dramatic when losing body fat.

Lean tissue includes blood, bones, muscles and vital organs. Losing lean tissue can be life-threatening and may even prevent normal functioning of the heart. Dr. Mary Ellen Sweeney of Emory University Medical School found that some women dieters lost heart muscle and the more severe the diet the more heart muscle was lost.

Losing lean tissue is not only dangerously unhealthy, but also contributes to an excessively "flabby" look while lowering caloric requirement and preventing an increase in metabolism.

How long does it take to increase metabolism?

Slight increases begin within one day but usually there is a definite noticeable increase within four to six weeks if the program has been followed in total. Some people who are highly motivated will follow the program very closely and will reap the benefits of increased energy as early as one to two days, which motivates them even more. This kind of person may increase the metabolism even faster. Allowing ample time for the metabolism to increase adequately is one of the reasons a "Binge Day" is added only after six weeks. By then, the metabolism has usually increased to a degree that the "Binge Day," if done properly, will not produce a weight gain.

Once the metabolism has been increased, do I go back to my old eating habits?

This program is designed to help you change your eating habits, and is *not* a diet that you go "on" and then "off" when you've lost weight. People who follow the beginning three to four weeks invariably adopt the new eating plan as part of their lifestyle. They like the new way they are eating, they are never hungry, they enjoy the increases in energy, their favorite foods are included, and they are losing weight permanently, not to mention the many health benefits.

If you return to old eating habits and become inactive, your metabolism will respond by slowing down again. Metabolism increases only to a normal rate. This should not be confused with a fast rate nor does it mean that you can constantly over-eat or eat high fat, high sugar "junk" foods every day. But, you will find that you can eat more food and even eat your "junk" foods *in moderation* once you reach your goal.

One of the primary goals of the program is to help you learn new eating habits to include favorite foods, that are not only enjoyable and healthy but will also increase metabolic functions for a lifetime.

3

THE DIETING MYTH

Dieting doesn't work! It doesn't work because it can't work! It can't work because it triggers an *increase* in body fat. Anyone who attempts to lose weight by dieting, is shifting gears to reverse in an attempt to go forward. The results are exactly opposite than those desired.

New research evidence is proving the errors of old dieting theories and is providing new information that makes weight control easier, healthier and permanent. In this chapter, I will discuss how dieting to lose weight causes an opposite effect, and actually *aggravates* problems with weight control.

The Dieting Trap

So predictable is the body's response to dieting, that failure can almost be guaranteed. The following sequence of familiar (to dieters) events illustrates the futility experienced by those who have attempted to diet away their excess pounds:

"D" day arrives ("D" for *Diet*). Motivation is usually high at the beginning of any new diet and is heightened even more by the success of the typical first week, when the pounds seem to be almost melting away (which is usually accounted for by the loss of fluid).

This feeling of accomplishment usually carries through the next few weeks even though the weight loss begins to slow down more with each passing week. Typically, after this slow down, a week or perhaps even two will follow when weight does not budge and without weight loss, motivation begins to dwindle. With determination, the dieter continues with the same number of calories, desperately hoping for a weight loss, but instead, begins to show a slight weight *gain*. Frustrated and puzzled, the dieter cannot understand the weight *gain* on the *same* food intake that produced a substantial weight *loss* the first few weeks. With stubborn persistence, another week is endured, only to bring another increase in weight. The dieter begins to ponder the hunger pangs, the calorie counting, the tasteless foods and wonders – for what? To gain weight? And so in frustration, the decision is made to end the diet. Upon returning to prior eating habits and foods, the weight is gained back more quickly than it was lost. The sad fact is that ultimately, the dieter ends up several pounds heavier than before dieting.

Dieting - 99.5% Failure

Overweight problems and dieting are on the increase, and it has been estimated that almost a third of our present American population is overweight. Most all dieters reported similar dieting failures with 99.5% failing to lose significant weight and/or maintain their weight losses. Researchers, prompted by the unbelievably high rate of failure, began investigating and found that the failures were not necessarily due to a lack of will power, but to the body's unique response to dieting.

Metabolism Lowered By Dieting

If you are overweight, chances are your metabolism is already slow. This means you are burning calories much slower than your thin friends. Dieting will slow your metabolism even more. When you cut back on your calorie intake, the body slows down its calorie burning rate. Why is this?

Before I can answer that question, let's take a brief look at the physiology and origins of some of the survival techniques adopted by the body in order to insure survival.

Humans have been on earth for over 2 million years, during which time frequent food shortages and famines proved a serious threat. The body responded to these food shortages by slowing down its rate of food burning – the metabolism, and "learned" to burn calories slower and more efficiently. As a result, early humans were able to survive long periods of time on the smaller amounts of food that were available and this slowing down of the metabolism became a survival technique to prevent starvation. When you go on a diet, you create an artificial food shortage and your body responds to the food shortage by slowing down the metabolism. Research has proven that if you lower your calorie intake, the body lowers its calorie burning rate to prevent starvation, just as it has been doing for over 2 million years!

But, you say, I know I'm not going to starve! *You* may know that, but your body responds to its immediate environment. For example, if it is 90 degrees in the shade outdoors, and you're sitting inside with the air conditioner set on 50 degrees, you'll soon start to shiver. Shivering is the body's first response to prevent freezing. *You* know you're not going to freeze – it's 90 degrees outside! But once again, your body responds to its immediate environment.

Whether a diet or a real food shortage, when calorie intake is lowered, the body responds by lowering its calorie burning rate.

After dieting, when returning to regular pre-diet eating habits, the metabolism is much lower, and weight is gained much faster than it was lost. Gradually, the metabolism begins to increase, but *not* back to its pre-diet rate! It will function at a slightly lower rate after each dieting attempt. For this reason, most people not only gain back the weight that was lost, but gain a few extra pounds more. It is estimated that because of this slightly lowered metabolism, there will be approximately 5% more weight gained back than was lost. If you were 200 pounds when you began dieting, this translates into an additional gain of 10 pounds to a total body weight of 210 pounds – an increase in weight brought on by dieting!

To make matters worse, a diet "teaches" your body to lower its metabolism so that with each dieting attempt, the metabolism declines even faster.

Illustration #3.1 is typical of the body's response to dieting.

Metabolism Lowered By Dieting

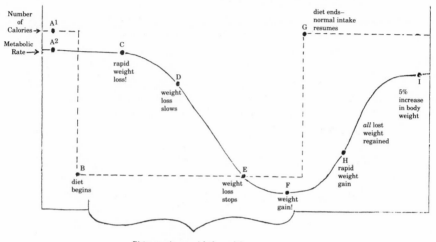

Dieter experiences weight *loss* and then weight *gain* on the *same number of calories*

A¹ & A² - Normal metabolic rate (A²) low; burn fewer calories than eaten (A¹).

B - Calorie intake decreased - low calorie diet begins.

C - Weight loss excellent – metabolism burning more calories than are being eaten.

D - Weight loss begins to slow down as metabolism begins to drop in response to lowered calorie intake.

E - Weight loss stops – metabolism burning same number of calories as are eaten.

F - Weight gain! Metabolism continues to drop until it is below calorie intake as seen at points A¹ & A².

G - Discouragement - diet ends and regular caloric intake is resumed as seen at A¹.

H - Rapid weight gain! Metabolism increasing slowly but is much slower than"normal".

I - Metabolism remains lower than before diet (A²). Weight is regained plus 5% more with mebabolism now slower (I) than before dieting (A²).

Chart #3.1

Fat Producing Enzymes Activated By Diet

Some of the enzymes produced by your body will increase fat production and fat storage. During a famine, these enzymes act like squirrels storing away nuts for the food shortage that winter brings, and will automatically become more active during a food shortage (diet) to increase storage of fat. Fat, in essence, is calories in storage and can be used by the body for fuel. One such fat-storing enzyme – adipose tissue lipoprotein lipase (AT-LPL) – increases in activity as much as four or more times as a result of dieting!

Brown Fat – The "Good" Fat

Brown fat is found in very small amounts around internal organs and between shoulder blades, and functions primarily to insulate internal body organs. This fat burns a tremendous number of calories to do its job of keeping the internal organs warm, especially during exposure to cold temperatures, and in this respect will assist with weight control.

Dieting has a negative effect on brown fat activity. In many studies, dieting decreased brown fat activity drastically, and in some cases to the point that there was no detectable brown fat activity at all!

Diets Sabotage Weight Loss

We must learn to work *with* the body, not at cross purposes. Dieting is not a natural state. It threatens the body's energy stores, causing automatic reactions that sabotage any weight loss you may have. Even worse, problems with weight control will only *increase* with each dieting attempt.

Low calorie diets do not supply enough food to insure an adequate intake of nutrients, especially protein. If dietary protein is inadequate, the body cannibalizes its own lean tissue, using it for its protein needs. This loss of lean tissue hampers dieting success because maintaining lean tissue requires extra calories. In fact, one reason men require more calories than women is because they have more lean tissue (muscle) than women. The *loss* of lean tissue will therefore *decrease* calorie requirements, which in turn will make weight loss more difficult.

Lean body tissue includes not only the muscles, but vital organs as well – heart, lungs, kidneys, etc. Repetitive dieting may result in an appreciable loss of lean tissue, causing a weakening of these organs, and in extreme cases, even death.

Chart #3.2 further illustrates the futility of dieting:

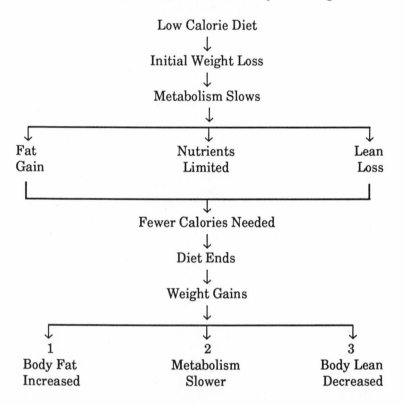

Fat storing enzymes (AT-LPL) – 4 or more times more active after Lo-Cal Diet.

Chart #3.2

Dieting Increases Fat and Weight

Extensive research has established the fact that dieting not only increases weight, but also alters body composition. An increase in body fat and a decrease in body lean typically follows a dieting attempt which in turn decreases the number of calories your body needs. Notice how body composition is changed and weight is increased in this typical "dieter":

(Spring) ON DIET Pounds Lost	(Fall) DIET ENDS Initial Pounds Regained	(Winter) FEW MONTHS LATER Total Pounds Regained
10 lbs. - fat	15 lbs. - fat	19 lbs. - fat
5 lbs. - lean	0 lbs. - lean	0 lbs. - lean
+5 lbs. - water	+5 lbs. - water	+6 lbs. - water
20 lbs.	20 lbs.	25 lbs.

1. Weight - increased 5 pounds
2. Body Fat - increased 9 pounds
3. Body Lean - decreased 5 pounds
4. Metabolism - slower
5. Caloric Requirement - lower

Almost twice as much fat has been regained by the above "dieter," while lean tissue has been decreased by 5 pounds! Research has found that the diet-induced slow-down in metabolism plus the increase in body fat and the decrease in body lean all contribute to a slowly increasing weight gain above pre-diet weight (see winter above). Each subsequent diet attempt produces a repetition of the same cycle with body weight steadily increasing from diet to diet. A few years and several dieting attempts later, this "dieting trap" will have victims gradually eating a little less, while gradually gaining a little more with each passing year.

All Diets Compound Weight Problems

Low calorie diets have been mentioned several times, and for clarification it must be stressed that any diet will produce the same end result. Diets compound weight problems primarily because of the slow down in metabolic functions.

While most diets restrict calorie consumption in one way or another, high protein diets are an exception. These diets severely restrict carbohydrates and require a high protein intake. Nevertheless, the end result is the same – a slow down in metabolic function. Here's how.

Working a little differently than low calorie diets, high protein diets have been shown to decrease thyroid activity. As little as a 10% decrease in thyroid activity reduces calories needed by several hundred per day. The thyroid gland secretes hormones that have a profound effect on the metabolic rate of the body. High protein diets *reduce* T_3, which is the active form of thyroid, and will also reduce the body's ability to burn calories, both of which will work to reduce metabolism.

Weight lost on high protein diets is very rapid and is also very misleading as it is mostly a water loss. Dehydrating the body, water is pulled from muscles and tissues to digest protein, leaving an estimated 1/3 less water in the body! Since 1/2 of body weight is water, a 150 pound person has 75 pounds of water, 1/3 of which (25 pounds) would be lost very quickly on a high protein diet. People are usually very elated with this tremendous "weight" loss which is actually a dehydration of their bodies. This is also the reason a high protein diet produces a very rapid *regain* – faster than any other dieting method. Stray from the high protein fare and dehydrated body tissues soak up water like a sponge, producing tremendous weight gains. In some cases as much as a 6-10 pound increase has occurred in just one day!

There are many health hazards associated with high protein dieting. In more than a few instances cardiac complications have occurred and in some cases have been severe enough to cause death. The diuretic effect of a high protein intake "leaches" minerals from the body that, while essential for all body functions, are especially critical for impulse transmission in the heart muscle. In addition, calcium loss reaches a dangerous level which cannot be prevented even with calcium supplements. As a result, bone density decreases contributing to osteoporosis, brittle bones, etc.

In the final analysis, it is clear that the frequent dieter actually increases weight problems and loses only one thing – good health!

Questions
The Dieting Myth

Why is it that every time I go on a diet, I lose weight in the beginning, but before long I stop losing and sometimes will even gain on the same number of calories?

Believe it or not, this is a common occurrence. To help you understand what is happening, let me first give you some background information.

For over two million years humans have existed on earth and food shortages and famines have been part of that existence. To prevent starvation the body "learned" to respond to these food shortages by slowing down the metabolism (food burning rate). This metabolic slow down is an automatic survival response which kept humans from becoming extinct, and will occur any time there is a food shortage, regardless of origin.

When you diet, you create an "artificial" food shortage and your body responds automatically by slowing down the metabolism to prevent starvation. During the first weeks of dieting with the metabolism just beginning to slow down you will lose weight because more calories are being burned than the smaller amount eaten. As the metabolism continues its gradual slow-down you will reach a point where calories are burned so slowly that you not only stop losing weight but begin to gain back some of the weight you've lost. In this instance your body is functioning in a totally normal manner, and has just successfully protected itself from what was interpreted as the beginning stages of starvation – a food shortage to the point that weight loss had begun to occur. Not understanding this you become perplexed and wonder what has gone wrong with your diet!

This is an example of the importance of understanding and working *with* your body and not at cross purposes, to achieve your desired weight goal. Research studies even with people of normal weight, show that dieting produces a decrease in metabolism, and at best, will produce only temporary weight loss.

I have dieted several times. At present I have just dieted back to 128 pounds. Why is it that I wear a size larger now than I did two years ago when I weighed exactly the same?

You indicate that you've lost weight several times which means you've also gained back the weight several times. Each dieting attempt alters body composition, increasing fat and decreasing lean tissue. Lean tissue is heavier and more compact, taking up less space, while body fat is lighter but takes up much more space. Dieting produces a loss of not only fat but also of lean tissue. When you gain back the weight, you gain only fat. In this manner there is an increase in fat which takes up more space than the lean tissue that was lost. For this reason, dieting to a previous weight will not necessarily return you to the same previous size. Losing lean tissue and regaining fat is much like replacing one pound of stones with one pound of feathers. While they both weigh one pound, the pound of feathers obviously will take up more *space* than the pound of stones.

Your body composition now includes more body fat, and as such, you will be larger at any given weight than previously.

I lose weight fast on a high protein diet. Is it really bad for your health?

Absolutely! Cardiac problems are not unusual in those who have gone on high protein diets, not to mention the adverse effects on thyroid activity which will slow down metabolism. Once again, this is another dieting approach and *diets don't work!*

Remember one very important fact about weight loss – "Fast" begins with "F" which stands for *Failure*! If anything promises extremely "fast" weight loss, you can be assured of subsequent failure!

What is the rationale of slow weight loss being best?

Your body can metabolize an average of 1-2 pounds of fat per week. If you increase the amount of your activity and follow the eating plan very strictly as suggested in "The Quick Weight Loss" plan, you will lose slightly faster. However, an extremely fast weight loss beyond the first week (when body fluid accounts for part of your weight loss) usually indicates that you're losing lean tissue which will spell disaster for keeping the weight off.

Ironic as it may seem, overweight people probably know more about *fast* weight loss than anyone else. Most of them can tell you several ways to lose it fast because they've done it fast many times over! Two things overweight people really need to know is 1) how to continue to lose to reach their goal, and 2) how to maintain that goal and not gain back what they've lost.

I remember as a fat person the word "fast" would catch my eye and my attention, quicker than anything else. Luckily I became a little wiser and realized I was already an expert at losing it *fast*! I changed my point of view and began looking for a way to lose it permanently.

What do you mean by the statement – "Diets don't work because they can't work"?

Each dieting attempt decreases lean tissue, increases body fat, decreases metabolism and decreases caloric requirements. Any *one* of these has the potential of halting weight loss. Dieting precipitates not *one*, but *all* of the above simultaneously, which renders continuing or permanent weight loss an impossibility!

4

CALORIES COUNT – OR _DO_ THEY?

In the laboratory, one calorie is that amount of energy required to raise one kilogram of water one degree Celsius. In the laboratory, calories act the same and it makes no difference what the time or what the source. But in the body, it makes a big difference! It is not possible to have laboratory controls in the body, and there are many variables at work that alter results.

Time – When and How Frequently You Eat Makes A Difference

Every time you eat, your metabolism increases. Extra calories are used to fuel all the many processes necessary to digest the food. This "heating up" effect after eating, is called the "thermic effect" of food and has some very important benefits.

First, this thermic effect requires extra calories, which means that some of the calories supplied by the food will be "lost" in production of heat. Second, the metabolism increases after eating requiring the body's use of calories at a much faster rate than normal throughout the entire digestive process. Therefore, every time you eat, the thermic effect of food and the increase in metabolism will increase your caloric expenditure. If you increase your *frequency* of eating with appropriate small between meal snacks you will increase your metabolism more frequently as well as the thermic effect. Thereby you will not only "waste" more calories but will convert fewer of them to fat. It is well known that people who eat four or more times per day are slimmer than those who eat three or fewer meals.

Eating more frequently will also help control your appetite. Remember how your mother told you not to eat between meals because it would "spoil" your appetite? With less appetite, there is less hunger at mealtimes and the tendency to over-eat is decreased. Over-eating is almost assured when you sit down to a meal ravenously hungry.

Your body produces less fat and more energy from smaller, frequent feedings. As a result, energy levels usually increase quickly, weight goes down, and the lethargic, "stuffed" feeling associated with eating too much does not occur.

Not only the frequency of eating, but the time of day you eat, will influence your body's fat production also.

Many people trying to lose weight will skip breakfast, eat a very light lunch, or none at all, and by evening, they are starving! They eat a large evening meal, which is their only meal of the day, and wonder why they aren't losing weight. If you're one of these people, you may be surprised to know that the *number* of calories is sometimes not as important as the way your body *uses* those calories! Here's why:

1. Going for long periods of time without food will cause the metabolism to begin slowing down – the body's automatic response to a food shortage, whether it's a real food shortage or one that you've created by not eating.

2. You've probably heard that evening eating will sabotage the most diligent attempt to lose weight. Two of the primary reasons are – first, the thermic effect of food is lower by evening, and second, your body's caloric requirements are lower by evening.

3. A large meal produces more body fat than smaller meals, eaten more frequently, even though the total daily caloric intake is the same. The large meal that leaves you feeling uncomfortably full supplies more calories than you need *at that time*. The body *stores* excess calories only one way – as fat! There are many interesting research studies that compare the effects of one meal a day versus smaller, frequent meals. Usually the small feedings produced a weight *loss*, but the same number of calories, all eaten in one large meal, produced a weight *gain*!

The following chart, #4.1, is designed to illustrate the possible differences in fat production by the *same* number of calories (1500), based on how they are eaten: 1) in three meals plus three snacks, or 2) in three meals with dinner the largest of the day. Eating three meals a day with the largest in the evening, is an American *custom*, based on convenience, not health. You came into this world (as an infant) eating 6 small feedings a day, a very healthy following of your natural, biological instincts. You were "trained," at a very early age, to eat three meals a day, which is so much more convenient! Convenient, yes, but at what price?

Calories From Dietary Fat Produce More Body Fat

Calories from high fat foods will produce more body fat than the same number of calories from low fat foods. Dietary fat is metabolically the easiest food for your body to convert to body fat. It has been said that when you spread the "mayo" on your sandwich, you may as well spread it on your hips! There may be more truth than jest in that statement! Here's how it works.

It is estimated that approximately 5% of the calories in fat foods are used for digesting these foods as compared to four times that number of calories, or 20%, for digesting carbohydrates and protein. For example, when you eat 600 calories of fat, only 5% (30 calories) are used for the digestive process, so you have *570* calories left for your fat cells. If you eat 600 calories of complex carbohydrate foods, your body has to work harder, using 20% (120 calories) for the digestive process leaving only *480* calories, some of which will not be absorbed because of the high fiber content of these foods. In comparison, both foods have the same number of calories (600) but after the digestive process your body actually gets 570 from fat and *less* than 480 from complex carbohydrates!

Chart #4.1

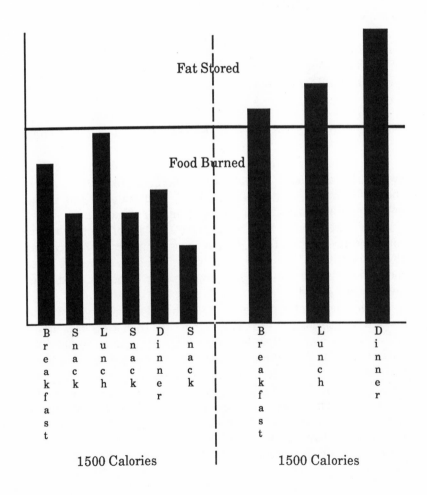

HOW THE BODY USES CALORIES
Meals and Snacks ————————————Three Meals

Fat Stored

Food Burned

| B r e a k f a s t | S n a c k | L u n c h | S n a c k | D i n n e r | S n a c k | B r e a k f a s t | L u n c h | D i n n e r |

1500 Calories   1500 Calories

Fiber Fights Fat!

Not only does a high fiber intake have many health benefits, but it will also aid in weight control. High fiber foods – grains, vegetables, etc. – will combine with the fat in a meal preventing some of its absorption, according to a United States Department of Agriculture report. Fiber also increases food transit time, which means that the fiber moves food through the intestines quicker, limiting caloric absorption. High fiber foods are usually very filling but not "calorie dense," and larger, more "filling" amounts may be eaten without a significant increase in caloric intake. For example, two small pieces of fudge take up a small space in your stomach as compared to three and a half baked potatoes, which have the same number of calories!

To aid in weight control, a high fiber food should be eaten with each meal and for snacks.

Simple and Complex Carbohydrates – There Is A Difference

"If I could only stay away from sweets . . . once I start eating sweets, I can't stop . . . I feel like I'm addicted to sweets . . ." Do these statements sound familiar? If so, your body's trying to tell you something about the carbohydrates you're eating.

There are two kinds of carbohydrates – *simple* and *complex*. Simple carbohydrate foods are easily remembered by associating the "s" in "simple" with the "s" in "sugar" and are primarily those foods that contain some form of simple sugar – desserts and other sweet tasting foods.

When the blood sugar level drops sharply, a strong desire for sweets is experienced – the body's message that it needs a "quick fix" to bring blood sugar levels back up as quickly as possible. Unfortunately, the simple carbohydrate (sweets) is very difficult for the body to handle and elevates blood sugar too high, too quickly. Having a simple molecular structure, simple carbohydrates are highly concentrated, and quickly absorbed, causing an abnormally sharp *rise* in blood sugar levels. This abnormal elevation precipitates an "over reaction" with the pancreas *oversecreting* insulin in such amounts that subsequently produces an abnormally sharp *drop* in blood sugar levels. This sharp drop again takes blood sugar levels *below* normal which will again create a craving for sweets (simple carbohydrate), causing another sharp rise, which in turn precipitates an oversecretion of insulin, which produces another sharp drop, and so the cycle is repeated. Many times this cycle begins with the omission of amino acids (protein) for breakfast, and is perpetuated throughout the day by simple carbohydrate foods, or a lack of complex carbohydrate foods.

The following chart, #4.2, illustrates typical blood sugar fluctuations produced by simple carbohydrate foods.

Chart #4.2

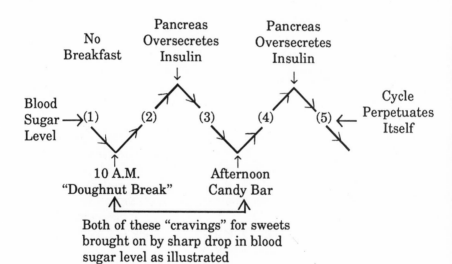

Both of these "cravings" for sweets
brought on by sharp drop in blood
sugar level as illustrated

1. Sharp beginning drop in blood sugar level precipitated by omitting *amino acids (protein)* at breakfast. This drop creates a craving for "sweets" - (doughnut).

2. Doughnut causes such a rapid rise that the body overreacts, oversecreting insulin which in turn causes a –

3. Rapid drop which again creates a craving for "sweets" – (candy bar) and the cycle is repeated. (4 & 5)

There are several things that are significant in these exaggerated fluctuations of the blood sugar level that will affect weight loss. First, energy levels fall dramatically when blood sugar levels fall, causing lethargy and inactivity. Second, when blood sugar levels fall sharply, the urge for "simple carbohydrates" (sweets) is almost uncontrollable. Eating them will cause a subsequent overproduction of insulin. Third, the excess insulin being secreted will cause an increase in fat production. *Insulin is a fat promoting hormone* and will encourage fat production and fat storage! Fourth, the fluctuations result in excessive insulin production. This, along with a weight gain and an increase in size of fat cells, causes these cells to become insulin-resistant. This resistance leads to a condition known as hyperinsulinism which is often a precursor to adult onset diabetes.

Because of the increased production of insulin initiated by simple carbohydrates, there is a greater increase in body fat than with the *same number of calories* from complex carbohydrates.

Found primarily in 1) vegetables, and 2) foods made from grains, complex carbohydrates have a more complex molecular structure and are absorbed much more slowly and evenly. As a result, blood sugar levels are stabilized, energy increases, and excess insulin production does not occur. Therefore, while calories are the same, simple carbohydrates affect the body differently than complex carbohydrates and as a result, will increase body fat *more*!

Complex carbohydrates also assist with the proper functioning of the thyroid, which plays a major role in weight control. Add to this the benefits of the high fiber content of complex carbohydrate foods, and it's easy to understand why this group of foods are a must for both health and weight control.

How The Body Uses Calories Is What Counts

All foods have calories — it's the kind of food and how each body *uses* the calories that counts. To say that a calorie behaves the same under laboratory conditions as in the body is as ridiculous as suggesting that if one gallon of gasoline produces 32 miles in laboratory tests, it will produce 32 miles in any kind of vehicle which, like humans, may vary from a Mack truck to a Volkswagen "beetle"!

In summary, the following dietary influences affect the way your body uses calories, and must be understood and considered in order for weight loss to be successful:

1. The thermic effect of food.

2. How often you eat.

3. When you eat (time of day).

4. Source of calories – fat, protein, complex or simple carbohydrates.

Questions
Calories Count Or Do They?

I always understood that calories are used for energy and an excess stored as fat. Is this information correct?

Partially. But the simplification of your statement omits some important facts. The calorie is needed to fuel every function of the body as long as you are alive. But there are variables to consider. Imagine a rheostat on a light switch. When it is turned up and the light is bright, more energy is used, but turned down, less energy is used and there are many variations of energy expenditures between high and low. Your body's energy expenditure is similar to the rheostat. There are certain situations when more energy is used and others when less energy is used. You use more calories earlier in the day than later in the evening. You use more calories to digest protein than you use to digest fat. Every time you eat, calorie expenditure increases to fuel the operation of digestion. When you perform certain kinds of activities, metabolism increases requiring a greater increase in calorie expenditure than if you were performing a different activity that used calories but did not increase metabolism. Eating in the earlier part of the day requires more calories to fuel the digestive processes than in the evening.

The bottom line is that we must become familiar with some of the basic physiological operations of our bodies. Then we will know not only when the "rheostat" is turned up but how to turn it up, so that most of the calories eaten will not contribute to fat, but to energy.

I am not suggesting a college degree in physiology. The basic principles discussed in this book are very simple, but are important and must be incorporated in any approach to weight control if it is to be permanent. In this respect, these principles are much like those of gravity – very simple, but so important that if you ignore them, you'll fall flat on your face!

You mean there are ways to make your body burn more calories?

Yes! 1) The more often you eat, the more often metabolism speeds up, using more calories. 2) Complex carbohydrates and proteins require more calories to digest than fats. 3) The thermic effect of food is greatest in the earlier hours of the day, which means that more breakfast and lunch calories will be "wasted" through this thermic effect than dinner calories. 4) Certain activities will increase metabolic rate and your fat-burning rate for 15-20 hours. (See Chapter - "Increase Fat Burning and Metabolism With A Daily Walk.")

Once I eat sweet foods, I seem to crave more. Why is this?

The insulin reaction to simple carbohydrates (sugary foods) causes a subsequent sharp drop in blood sugar levels which precipitates a strong craving for more sweets to elevate this abnormally low level, a reaction which is repeated, and thus perpetuates itself. (See chart#4.2 in this Chapter).

I had cake and ice cream at a birthday party last evening. This morning I was surprised when I showed a 2 pound gain! How can I gain weight like this in only one day?

Your 2 pound gain is not a true weight gain. Sweets produce an increase in body fluid retention. Many people are surprised when they notice swollen hands or feet the next day after having sweets, because we assume that only sodium causes water retention.

Never weigh yourself the morning after having sweets. Wait two or three days to allow fluid retention to dissipate and then your weight will be more accurate. It would be next to impossible to gain two pounds of fat in one day!

Are you saying that not all carbohydrates are good for you?

Not for weight loss. There are two kinds of carbohydrates – simple and complex. The simple ("s" in "simple" stands for "sugar") are the fat producers because of their caloric density and also because of the insulin reaction they produce (see chart). Complex carbohydrates (vegetables and anything made from grains) assist with proper functioning of the thyroid, are not calorie dense, and produce satiety without excess calories. They also help stabilize blood sugar levels, keeping energy levels high.

Are you suggesting that I stop counting calories?

Absolutely! Eat until you are comfortable (never hungry, never stuffed), limit fat and sugar intake and *forget calories*! If you are going to count anything, count fat grams. This does not mean you should get bogged down counting *all* fat grams, since even fruits and vegetables contain some fat. Limit *obvious* fat sources such as meats, nut butters, margarine, etc., to 20-25 grams daily. Also, get into the habit of reading food labels if you buy already prepared foods.

Which foods do you recommend for a good source of fiber?

Complex carbohydrate foods are also high in fiber – vegetables and foods made from grains. Also, some fruits are high in fiber. Probably one of the best foods for insoluble fiber is unprocessed bran. Quaker puts out an unprocessed bran that is available in most supermarkets. People having problems with constipation usually respond very well with the addition of 3-4 tablespoons of unprocessed bran each morning to their hot or cold cereal because of the high fiber content.

I've heard a lot about fiber helping to control weight. How does this work?

There are two different kinds of fiber – soluble and insoluble. Both are excellent in improving health, with soluble fiber being especially beneficial in reducing blood cholesterol in some people. Insoluble fiber is especially beneficial in weight control. It gives a "full" feeling without a lot of calories, increases food transit time, and prevents the absorption of some of the fat in food.

5

SUPPLEMENTS TO ENHANCE HEALTH AND WEIGHT LOSS

Using nutritional supplements is a very controversial issue. Most books on weight control may briefly mention using a vitamin/mineral supplement and quickly move on to another topic as if they're handling a hot poker! They purposely do not dwell on this controversial subject, and I can understand why.

I must admit that I had my doubts about including recommendations for supplements, wondering if such a controversial subject would detract from the credibility of my book. After pondering for some time, I decided I must include information on the two supplements, amino acids and vitamin/minerals I recommend to all my "Fat To Fit" participants. I realized that controversial or not, the success of these people, as well as my own, has been phenomenal and using these two supplements has definite benefits.

I am not suggesting that the program's success depends entirely upon their use, but I do know that using these supplements will certainly assist in producing weight loss and enhancing health. I've seen it happen hundreds of times in people I've worked with in the past and those I am working with now. I recommend that the detailed information about the benefits of their use be read, and then the decision to use these supplements be based on past dieting attempts and eating habits.

Are Supplements Necessary?

Ideally, all nutrients should come from food alone, and when no food is refined, and all are grown in nutrient-rich, chemical-free soils and eaten within a short period of time from harvest, supplements may not be necessary. In today's world, this is not possible, and supplements are not only essential to good health, but will also assist in normalization of body weight. Supplements are nothing more than nutrients that would have been furnished in food were it of excellent quality. They are too often mistakenly viewed as drugs because they are made up in pill or capsule form. It is as erroneous to consider sugar cubes a drug after they have been extracted from their natural source and pressed into a "cube" form as it is to consider amino acids or vitamins as drugs after being extracted from their natural source and made into tablet form. It is interesting to note that a recent survey of dieticians who stated emphatically that supplements were definitely not necessary, were, themselves, using dietary supplements. Taking supplements is not "treating disease" but is insuring optimum health and weight normalization. It must be remembered that medicine is the study of disease; nutrition, the study of health; medicine is primarily curative; nutrition primarily preventive.

Nutrient Requirements and RDA's

The RDA (Recommended Dietary Allowance) is a recommended estimate based on the *average* individual of *average* size, *average* health, and *average* activity. Ironically, there is *no average* individual, because there are no two bodies that are exactly alike. The combination of genes you inherit from your parents that determines your physical characteristics, etc., is a combination that is uniquely yours and is never reproducible. A surgeon or a surgical nurse sees the insides of many bodies and they will be the first to tell you that not even body organs such as gall bladders, kidneys or lungs, are ever exactly the same, but are different sizes, colors and locations. Notice the variety in eyes, hair, noses, skin – none are exactly the same. Some persons are more energetic, while there are some who are more lethargic. An average person does not exist. So a hypothetical estimate based on a hypothetical "average" is useless! Each person is different, eats differently, and is exposed to different mental and physical stresses, all of which affect their nutrient requirements.

Some Known Nutrient Deficiencies

It is common knowledge that many American women have insufficient iron in their diets. To compound the problem, there are several dietary and medicinal substances which "block" the body's absorption of the already insufficient amount of iron. Our ever increasing consumption of antacids decreases iron absorption substantially. Tea (tannic acid) also decreases iron absorption. Even if the dietary iron intake is adequate, it does not necessarily insure adequate iron absorption for the body's use.

Women using oral contraceptive agents are highly susceptible to folic acid (a B vitamin) deficiency. Folates in food are easily destroyed by storing, cooking, and other processing. With our modern technology of food storage and processing, this nutrient is easily destroyed.

Zinc is an essential mineral and is involved in almost every bodily function. Many studies are showing marginal states of zinc deficiencies in Americans, because of zinc deficient soils in which our foods are grown. A zinc deficiency may also be caused by a diet of highly refined foods, especially simple carbohydrates (American diets?). Because of refining processes, zinc is almost totally lacking from white sugar, white flour, and all products made from these two ingredients.

Acne is being treated by some medical doctors, with zinc and vitamin A since it is felt that acne may be caused principally by a zinc deficiency.

Pyridoxine, or B_6 is one of several of the B complex vitamins, and is essential for many things that contribute to good health.

Antibiotics and some sulfa drugs destroy vitamin B_6 in the body, and in food. B_6 is destroyed by long periods of storage, chemicals and light. All the B complex vitamins are essential for good health and are totally safe since there is no toxic effect even in relatively large doses.

The above are just a few examples, as the list of altered or destroyed nutrients in our modern American diets appears to be increasing. There is no question in the minds of nutrition professionals who keep abreast of current nutrition research, that supplementation is essential to good health. In our modern culture there have been many advances in food technology, but we must remember that this can be a double-edged sword. Technology has helped increase production, supply and convenience, but with a price. It is true that we no longer have widespread food shortages in our country, and we have many conveniences including super market shopping and fresh produce all year long. But, we pay a price − a decrease in the health supporting nutrients and an increase in additives in our food supply.

Dieting compounds nutrition problems and most people do not realize the dangers involved. Dieting means food restriction and food restriction means nutrient restriction. People who have a history of dieting may unknowingly have weakened hearts because of protein loss, or other health problems because of nutrient deficiencies promoted by these diets.

A suggested part of this program to maintain or increase health, and to assist with weight control, is the use of an elemental yield vitamin/mineral supplement and amino acid supplements, both of which are discussed briefly in the remainder of this chapter.

Amino Acids

It is believed that man has been on planet Earth for over 2 million years. For most of that time, his protein needs were supplied by the very lean meats of wild animals. Today our dietary meats are quite different. Our farm animals are not running wild but are purposely fattened for slaughter and the meat reaching our tables is higher in fat than ever before. Essential amino acids are food elements in protein that are required to support life, but the fat in that same food is killing us. However, lowering protein intake to decrease dietary fat will also decrease amino acid intake. Conversely, increasing protein intake to insure an adequate supply of amino acids will *increase* dietary fat.

How can we get these necessary basic elements of life, the amino acids, without a high intake of dietary fat? The answer is simple. Decrease protein intake to a moderate level which will decrease dietary fat and add amino acid supplements. This will assist in both weight loss and health benefits. These supplements are amazingly effective, yet free of dangerous side effects.

What Are Amino Acids?

Amino acids are food elements and are the basic components of protein. Probably the most important nutrients needed by the body, amino acids are supplied by protein foods.

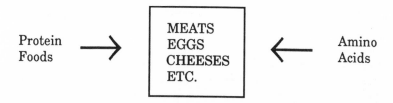

Proteins include lean meat, fish, poultry, seafoods, milk and milk products, as well as plant sources—beans and peas, breads, pastas, nuts and nut butters. For simplicity, only the primary sources have been included in the illustration.

The primary importance of including protein foods in the diet is to supply the necessary life supporting amino acids. A certain number of grams of protein are required simply to insure the proper intake of amino acids. Calculating grams of protein is easier and more efficient than calculating amino acids, but nevertheless, it is the amino acid requirement that we are speaking of when we talk about the body's protein requirements. Therefore, the body's protein needs are actually the body's amino acid needs. So important are the amino acids it contains, if just *one* of the essential amino acids is missing, that food is called "incomplete" protein.

Why Are Amino Acids Important?

There are so many functions of amino acids that it would take an entire book to discuss them all. However, for our purposes, let's look briefly at just a few.

Amino acids are necessary for stabilizing blood sugar levels, an extremely important function, and especially so for weight control. Many "sugar urges" are brought on by a drop in blood sugar levels, which will occur without adequate amino acid intake, most noticeably at breakfast. In fact, the practice of having coffee and doughnut breaks at mid-morning is not just a weakness for sweets, but is most likely the result of a blood sugar drop precipitated by a lack of amino acid intake at breakfast. It is interesting to note that most overweight people are not breakfast eaters and if they have a craving for sweets, these "sugar urges" may well be due to their lack of amino acid intake, especially at breakfast.

Along with amino acids, complex carbohydrates play an important role in stabilizing blood sugar levels also, and are discussed in another chapter. If you are one of those people who crave sweets, be sure to read this chapter.

Amino acids are essential for life. Life cannot be supported without amino acids. Most all bodily functions, from increasing energy and endurance to lean tissue production for firming and toning your body, are directly dependent upon your amino acid intake.

Amino Acids Help Reduce Body Fat

This property of amino acids has been exploited and some less than reputable vitamin companies are suggesting you can sit back in your easy chair, take amino acid tablets and lose weight. This is definitely not the case! Amino acids do however have a positive effect on basal metabolism, which in simple terms, determines the rate at which you use food for all bodily processes including energy production. If the metabolism is slow, less of the food eaten is used for energy, which means more will be stored as fat. The primary objective in weight control is to increase the metabolism so as to use more food for energy, and store less as fat. Amino acids are very effective in helping normalize the slow metabolism in over-weight people, when used in conjunction with the suggested eating and activity plans.

Amino acids also help reduce body fat by contributing to an increase in energy levels, which in turn precipitates an automatic increase in movement and activity. The tired, sluggish individual tends to sit as much as possible and move as little as possible in an attempt to rest – to conserve what little energy there is and thereby automatically uses fewer calories in day to day activities. A higher level of energy automatically precipitates more movement. Think about a time when you have felt tired and sluggish – how you tended to sit as much as possible, move as little as possible in order to rest – to conserve your energy and as a result, you used fewer calories in your daily activities. Compare this with a time when you felt energetic – you automatically move more, sit less, and engage in more activity, all of which increases your body's caloric expenditure. Therefore, amino acids will help reduce body fat by normalizing metabolism as well as increasing energy.

Peptide Bond and Free Form Combination Amino Acids

A pharmaceutical grade *peptide bond and free form* combination amino acid supplement is the only amino acid supplement the body uses effectively. Extracted from protein in a totally natural process, using pancreatic enzymes, these amino acids are in the only form that the body can use efficiently and safely. Unfortunately there are companies looking more at profit than health, who produce an inferior and useless product by using alkaline or acid chemicals to extract the amino acids from protein. The resulting amino acids cannot be utilized by the body and are excreted. Also, amino acids that are sold as "free form" alone, are not utilized properly and may cause serious side effects with prolonged use.

Vitamin/Mineral Supplements

Along with a peptide bond, free form combination amino acid supplement, I also recommend a second supplement – an elemental yield vitamin/mineral. A vitamin/mineral that is an elemental yield is one that is made from the nutrients themselves, so that the potencies listed on the label of the container are accurate. Vitamins that are not elemental are processed differently and nutrient potency may be quite different than the label states. An elemental yield vitamin/mineral supplement is simply one of higher quality and more accurate potency. Sometimes "elemental yield" appears on the label, sometimes not. If a supplement does not state "elemental yield" on the label, request a "truth of disclosure" from the manufacturer. If this is not possible, the only reliable way to find out is to have an analysis of the product done by an independent laboratory, which is very costly.

Unfortunately, there are many inferior products on the market due to the fact that quality control and regulation of food supplements is not adequate. Many companies sell and distribute supplements that they know little or nothing about, except their marketability and profit margin. Most of these supplements would be best flushed down the toilet!

Look for a reputable company that sells quality products and employs health professionals who know their products thoroughly and can offer services in assisting with proper choice and use of their products. I am keenly aware of individuals who fall prey to the "hard sell" approach and purchase supplements that are promised to do everything from growing hair on bald heads to "burning fat" off of fat people! This is unfortunate, as it reflects negatively on the reputable companies that are helping us become more health conscious.

It should be noted here, that mega doses of supplements are never to be used unless recommended by a physician who keeps you under close supervision. "If a little helps – more is better" is definitely not the case! Many people are using high-dosage vitamin preparations for various alleged benefits from youth restoration, to prevention of heart disease and cancer. These reports are frequently not based on scientific evidence. Self-treatment with high dosages of vitamins is dangerous and toxicity is a real threat to good health.

Participants in the "Fat to Fit" program use supplements in moderation – amino acids, to reduce dietary fat intake, and a vitamin/mineral supplement to insure health benefits. Those who have been hypertensive, diabetic, hypoglycemic, as well as those with elevated blood cholesterols and triglycerides, have had especially impressive health benefits along with their weight losses.

Use amino acids and vitamin/mineral supplements only as suggested. Using more than moderate amounts will be counter productive unless your physician suggests that you do so, based on your body chemistry profile!

Once again, it must be noted here that while amino acid supplements are highly recommended, they are not absolutely necessary and the program will work without them. However, it has been my experience in working with "Fat to Fit" participants that it is easier, healthier and more effective in reducing body fat if they are included.

Questions
Supplements To Enhance Health and Weight Loss

I have asked my doctor on several occasions about nutrition and supplements. Can I trust his suggestions?

Weight control, proper eating and use of supplements are all part of nutrition, which is preventive medicine – a relatively new concept. Doctors who have been practicing medicine for longer than five years probably did not receive nutrition education because it was either not included, or included only minimally in their medical schools. The American Medical Association is reportedly urging more nutrition education in medical schools. In the meantime, ask your doctor if he/she has been to seminars or taken extra classes on nutritional science. If they have not, get your nutritional advice elsewhere. All public libraries carry many nutrition books, some of which are written by doctors who have gone primarily into the study and practice of nutrition. But do be careful! Some of these books may be very confusing, and since nutrition is such a new science, you will find one author may contradict another. It is difficult at this time to get totally unbiased, scientific, and accurate information on nutrition.

Is there any legitimate, reliable research indicating a need for supplements?

Yes! Many! Here are just a few:

- Jeanine Barone, nutritionist and exercise physiologist with the American Health Foundation, a research group in New York, says that many Americans eat less than the RDA for zinc. Zinc is an essential mineral and is involved in more than 70 enzyme reactions.

- Research has proven a zinc deficiency may be involved in significant declines in immunity.

- Recent studies show that zinc gluconate helps reduce the incidence and severity of common colds.

- Studies show that Vitamin C supplements may decrease the severity of colds, has inhibited some tumors in animals and for the smoker is an absolute necessity.

- Research has shown that Vitamin E supplements lowered infections in laboratory animals who were exposed to bacteria.

- There are many research studies that show inadequate iron intake among Americans and almost as many showing an inadequate intake of some of the B vitamins and some essential minerals.

- Dr. Robert Haas in his book *Eat to Win* says that his research in nutritional supplementation demonstrates that active people improve their health, endurance and energy levels with nutritional supplements.

- The American Academy of Pediatrics says that today's children are definitely less fit. Only 10%, nationwide, are able to pass the Presidential Fitness Test designed for school children of all ages.

Once again let me caution you that more is not better! Use an elemental yield vitamin/mineral supplement and do not exceed the dosage suggested on the label. Large amounts of vitamin/mineral supplements are not recommended.

Should I take vitamin/mineral supplements every day?

I feel it is best to skip two days a week, so the vitamin/mineral supplements will be used more effectively. Your body tends to build a tolerance to anything you take on a regular basis, same amount, same time, over and over again every day. Skipping two days, such as the weekend, will avoid this and the vitamin/mineral supplement will remain much more effective.

I have read that if you are healthy and if your diet is adequate, supplements are not necessary. How valid is this?

I don't like to answer a question with a question, but in this case I feel I must. 1) How many Americans eat an "adequate" diet? 2) What is "adequate"? 3) What is "healthy"? 4) Consider just one nutrient, zinc, an essential mineral. Much of our American soil is zinc deficient. This means our crops will be zinc deficient, and our livestock eating the zinc-deficient crops grown on these soils will be zinc deficient. If this is the case, where will we get food – animal or plant, that will supply an adequate intake of zinc?

I find it very interesting that without criticism, our "winning" race horses get an average of 32 supplements, "winning" show dogs 35 supplements and similar amounts are fed to our farm animals, mink, fox, and many of our household pets. Not only is it an accepted practice to use supplements for these prized animals, but most of these supplemental mixtures are superior to any sold for humans. You can rest assured that these animals never get "fast foods," prepared mixes, sugary cereals, or any of the hundreds of other low nutrient, high fat foods sold for human consumption. Do we value the health of our animals more than that of our own, or our children?

Our food technology has given us great variety and convenience as far as our food choices are concerned. However, this same technology is also responsible for the reduction of many nutrients in our modern day foods. The extra processing, longer shipping and storage times, plus use of chemical fertilizers, insecticides, as well as the practice of early harvesting before maturity gives us tremendous increases in food yield and convenience, but at the same time has adverse effects on many essential nutrients in our foods.

Biochemist Paul Saltman, Ph.D, at the University of California, San Diego, chief author of *The California Nutrition Book* (Little & Brown) and leader of the University of California group that wrote "The New Nutrition" course for UCSD and *American Health* magazine is an advocate of supplements in our diets. Dr. Saltman feels that we must avoid excess fat, eat a variety of foods and use supplements to insure adequate intake of nutrients that may be lacking in our meals.

Patricia Hausman, author of *The Right Dose: How To Take Vitamins and Minerals Safely* (Rodale Press) reported her feelings about the supplements debate in a recent issue of *American Health* magazine. She believes the stand against the use of supplements taken by some of our health professionals is based on opinion, not on scientific fact and is therefore not in our best interest. I totally agree with this view!

The statement that we don't need supplements if we are "healthy" and eating an "adequate" diet is a vague, questionable "catch-all" statement used by those who perhaps lack adequate knowledge of much of the recent research dealing with supplements and the nutrition sciences.

What is meant by "incomplete" and "complete" protein?

Amino Acids are to protein what the alphabet letters are to words. There are many amino acids and many different combinations which make up a great variety of proteins. Every amino acid is not in each protein just as every letter of the alphabet is not in each word.

There are approximately twenty-two commonly occurring amino acids in our foods. The body can produce all but ten. These ten are called "essential" amino acids because our bodies cannot produce them and it is essential they be provided in our dietary intake. (Opinions vary as to the number of essential amino acids from eight to nine to ten.)

If a protein food is lacking in one or more of the essential amino acids, it is called "incomplete protein" – a protein the body cannot use. The amino acids will be deaminized and excreted.

The ratio of one amino to the other is equally important. If the intake of any one of the essential amino acids is too low, most of the others will not be used but will be deaminized and the nitrogen excreted leaving the body in a negative nitrogen balance. Life cannot be supported in a negative nitrogen balance and if continued, death will ensue.

A protein supplying all of the essential amino acids in the right ratio and in significant amounts so as to supply completely the amino acid needs of the body is called a "complete" protein. Meat, fish, seafood, poultry, milk, eggs, and cheeses are complete proteins having high biological values. A word of caution – it is not totally accurate to say that amino acids are either essential or non-essential. They are ALL needed in proper balance to support good health and a longer more productive life.

Isn't it possible to get all the needed amino acids from food?

Yes, most definitely! But, with high quality protein as the best food source of amino acids, you most likely will also get a high intake of fat (meat, eggs, cheese, milk). It is for this basic reason that I recommend a moderate protein intake along with the use of amino acid supplements.

Couldn't I stop eating protein food, substitute amino acids and lower my fat intake even more?

It would lower your fat intake, but unless you are truly dead set on being a strict vegetarian, I would recommend that you not omit protein food totally. There are other nutrients in protein food that will enhance health.

On a low fat intake, why not substitute amino acids for beef?

First of all most people like beef and it is important that you modify and do *not* omit any food that you like. Omitting foods you like will almost insure failure and you will feel deprived. Deprivation will eventually lead you back to old eating habits in order for you to enjoy your favorite foods.

Second, it is a fact proven through research that no matter who it is – the overweight, the diabetic, the heart patient, etc., food restriction always leads to overindulgence!

Third, beef is a good source of important nutrients, especially zinc and iron that are essential to good health. Therefore, if you like beef eat it lean and modify your intake to once or twice a week.

I don't like taking pills! Is it absolutely necessary to take amino acids?

No! I recommend amino acid supplements for reasons stated previously, especially to keep fat intake low without compromising amino acid intake. However, it must be your decision whether or not to use them.

Is there something I can substitute for the amino acids suggested on the menus?

Yes. Three to four hard boiled egg whites, or 2/3 cup of low-fat cottage cheese or 2/3 cup of fat-free yogurt – any one of these three may be substituted wherever you see amino acid tablets on the menu.

Are there other health benefits of amino acids other than those you've discussed?

Many! There are whole books that have been written about the benefits and importance of amino acids. One that is especially good for the lay person is Carlson Wade's, *Amino Acids Book.*

Recently, the Associated Press reported that researchers at the National Institutes of Health in Bethesda, Maryland found that a laboratory synthesized peptide (a compound made up of amino acids) proved to be highly successful as a cancer fighter. In experiments with rats who were injected with lung cancer cells, the researchers reported that those who were given the amino acid compound developed *no* lung cancer, while the rats not receiving the amino acid compound developed an average of fifty-one lung tumors!

This is not to suggest that you should take amino acids to prevent cancer, but it is an excellent example of the progress being made with use of these nutrients in health care.

Slowing the aging process, enhancing metabolic processes, hormone, antibody and enzyme formations, rejuvenating skin, hair and nails, soothing depression, increasing energy and even boosting sexual desire are only a few of the great number and variety of contributions made by a properly balanced intake of amino acids. They are fundamental to every living material, to the basic composition of every cell in the body and are the key not only to health but to life itself.

Can you take too many amino acid supplements?

You can take too much of anything. Your body will only use what it needs. Why waste your money? For example, if eating one tomato is good for you, does that mean eating 100 tomatoes is even better? Absolutely not! Eating 100 tomatoes would produce some very uncomfortable side effects including a grandiose stomach upset and diarrhea!

Some of the professional and world class athletes I've worked with may use as many as 30-35 amino acid tablets daily, but they are performing at extremely high intensity levels, requiring an increase of all nutrients.

For weight loss, use of amino acid supplements is beneficial in that protein food intake may be reduced to help lower fat intake. They will also assist in increasing metabolic functions, regulating blood sugar levels and increasing energy levels. Only the moderate amounts recommended are necessary to achieve these benefits.

Why is it important to use a blend of "pharmaceutical grade peptide bond and free-form" amino acid supplements?

When you eat protein food, digestion breaks down the protein into amino acids with chemical linkages called "peptide bonds" and some free form amino acids, all of which are absorbed from the intestine. This is a natural process and one that is duplicated by using natural pancreatic enzymes to break down a protein (for instance, casein from milk) into its amino acid constituents, which are used in producing a pharmaceutical grade peptide bond free-form amino acid supplement. This natural source and process used to produce amino acid supplements is essential in insuring an end product that is an exact replica of the end product of the body's natural processing of protein into amino acids. This will insure efficient, healthful use as the body, with unerring accuracy, will assemble these amino acids into vital substances needed.

There are other much cheaper processes that are used to produce amino acids but not in a natural form. As such, they will not be utilized properly by the body and in most cases may cause serious side effects when used for prolonged periods of time. "Peak" is a brand I've had analyzed and usually recommend to anyone who wishes to use amino acid supplements.

How do you feel about "one-a-day" vitamin/mineral supplements?

If it is only a "one-a-day" tablet, I question whether it is an elemental yield supplement unless the potency is very low. There are many vitamins and minerals listed on the labels of most of the "one-a-day" vitamins I've seen. If claims are made of a high potency formula in just *one* tablet, it would conceivably be almost the size of a golf ball! More importantly, supplements are concentrated food components. I feel the body can use them more efficiently if spaced throughout the day, with meals, rather than taking a full day's supply all at one time.

6

INCREASE FAT BURNING AND METABOLISM WITH A DAILY WALK

To most overweight people, "exercise" is a dirty word. Considering the routines of most exercise classes, I can't say I blame them. Even the word "exercise" conjures up thoughts of kicking the legs or rolling the arms until they're ready to drop off! Unfortunately, this "no pain, no gain" idea that has been instituted by many fitness instructors is totally erroneous, and often produces results that aren't worth the effort. These exhaustive exercises may have some conditioning benefits and on TV many of them are even entertaining. But for the average fitness-minded person, the idea of working to the limit is not the best approach and for the overweight person, is next to impossible.

When it comes to weight control, the most efficient activities for producing maximum fat burning and increased metabolism are quite simple. In fact, you will burn more fat just taking a brisk walk than you will by sweating through most so-called "aerobics" classes! Let me explain.

To increase fat burning and metabolism, an activity must include three essential aspects: 1) exercise heart rate, 2) adequate amount of time, and 3) an increase in maximum oxygen uptake

(VO2 max). If the activity meets these three requirements, it is called "aerobic." Unfortunately, most exercise classes are not designed properly to produce an increase in maximum oxygen uptake (number 3). They may be called "aerobic" classes, but they are definitely not aerobic!

These classes may work you to the limit of endurance, and they will burn calories from glucose or glycogen, but they *won't* cause your body to start breaking down fat stores. The task of burning fat is left to aerobic activities, which not only decreases the body's fat stores, but will also increase your metabolic rate. Aerobic activity produces an increase in fat burning and metabolism not only during the activity, but for approximately 15-20 hours *after* the activity is over! The extension of these benefits beyond the actual activity is still another reason body fat is lost much faster.

There are a variety of aerobic activities, but to start your program, I suggest walking or rebounding on the mini trampoline. There are many reasons that I feel these are the best activity choices.

Almost anyone in reasonable health can walk or use a "mini tramp." Both of these activities are easy to perform, do not require large investments of money, are safe, convenient, and enjoyable. Many people do both activities, while some prefer walking and use the mini tramp as an option on rainy days or when other inclement weather conditions exist. Either way, these activities will give quick and dependable results in increasing metabolism and fat burning.

Make no mistake, *the eating plan* and *the activity plan* must be used *together*! One will not work without the other. Choose one of the activities, or for variety, alternate the two, but whatever your choice, your activity must be a *daily priority*.

The Best Time For Activity

The best time of day to do your activity is in the morning. Research has shown that the body uses the same number of calories doing the activities in the morning as in the evening, but 2/3 of those calories come from body fat in the morning, and less than half the calories come from body fat in the evening. Getting up a little earlier in the morning will give you a special time planned without interruption for your activity.

However, if this is not possible, the second best time is in the evening, right before dinner, which has special benefits also. The metabolism will be increased when you eat your evening meal after your activity. Also, the activity initiates the production of a hormone that is both an appetite depressant and a mood elevator. With increased metabolism and less appetite, the evening meal will produce less body fat.

Instructions on how to begin and how to increase your activity, either walking or using the mini trampoline, will be discussed briefly in the next few paragraphs followed by a more detailed level by level plan at the end of this chapter.

Mini Trampoline

If you prefer to do your daily activity indoors, the "mini tramp" is for you. In the very beginning put your mini tramp in front of a mirror. Watching yourself helps with balance. Later when you feel comfortable with your balance, place it in front of the TV and watch your favorite program as you jog in place or jog to the rhythm of music you like on radio or cassette tape. Begin with five minutes jogging in place and swing your arms slightly. Increase your time gradually as you feel comfortable (see "Mini Trampoline – How To Begin") until you reach 50-60 minutes non-stop at your exercise heart rate (see chart #6.1). Always begin slowly, warming up for at least 4 minutes and checking your heart rate every 15-20 minutes. Don't rush it. It may take 4-6 weeks or longer to comfortably increase your time to 50-60 minutes. Once you have reached 30 minutes non-stop, check with the fitness club in your area and see if aerobic classes performed on mini trampolines are offered. Take these classes for fun and variety – you'll enjoy them! Aerobic classes done on the floor cannot be recommended because of the increasing number of injuries plus the fact that most are not totally aerobic.

Mini Trampoline – How To Begin

1. Gentle bounce or step in place 4 minutes. (warm up)

2. Jog in place 3 minutes – get off trampoline and walk around room 2 minutes – alternate 3 minutes on and 2 minutes off the tramp for a total of 30 minutes. When you can do 30 minutes comfortably, begin to increase (see below). Check EHR (Exercise Heart Rate) every 10 minutes.

3. Walk around the room for 5 minutes. (cool-down)

4. Stretch (see chapter on stretching for illustrations).

Note – If you have never used a mini tramp before, place it in front of a mirror, begin with an easy bounce *without* picking feet up off the mini trampoline. When you feel comfortable with your balance, begin picking up your feet and "march" in place, then jog slowly in place. When comfortable with this, swing your arms and bring your knees up slightly higher as you jog in place. *Do not begin above sequence until you feel comfortable with your balance.*

Mini Trampoline – How To Increase

1. Continue sequence above (#1-4) and begin gradual 10 minute increases in *total* time, alternating on and off the trampoline as in step #2 to a total of 60 minutes, which is your goal.

2. When you can comfortably do 60 minutes, alternating jogging on the trampoline, and getting off the trampoline to walk, gradually decrease 2 minute walking intervals to 1 minute; to 1/2 minute; then eliminate walking intervals *totally*. Check EHR every 15 minutes.

3. *Never* eliminate #1 warm up, #3 cool down, and #4 stretch. It is important that these *always* be included with each activity!!

Fast Walk

If your preference is the out-of-doors, fast walking is an excellent activity for you. Begin with a 4 minute "stroll" to warm-up, then gradually begin walking as fast as you comfortably can, taking long strides, swinging your arms and alternating 3 minutes of fast walking and 2 minutes of "strolling" for a total of 30 minutes. Gradually increase to 60 minutes, walking 30 minutes one way and then walking back 30 minutes.

Always begin with a warm-up "stroll" of 4 minutes. Check EHR at 15 minute intervals. You may want to buy an inexpensive child's watch with a second hand to check EHR, if you don't already have one. On rainy days or when there are other inclement weather conditions, do your activity indoors on a mini trampoline.

Fast Walk – How To Begin

1. 4 minutes stroll. (warm-up)

2. 3 minutes *fast walk and 2 minutes stroll – alternate these two for a total of 20-30 minutes. Check EHR every 15 minutes.

3. 5 minutes stroll. (cool-down)

4. Stretch (see chapter on stretching for illustrations).

* Be sure to take long strides and swing arms when doing *fast walk* after warm-up (#1).

Fast Walk – How To Increase

1. Continue sequence (#1-4, "How To Begin") and begin gradual 10 minute increases in step #2 to a total of 60 minutes.

2. When you can comfortably do 60 minutes, alternating fast and slow, begin to *decrease* 2 minute stroll intervals gradually to 1 minute; to 1/2 minute; then eliminate stroll intervals *totally* so

that you are walking fast for the entire 60 minutes. Check EHR every 20 minutes.

3. *Never* eliminate #1 warm-up, #3 cool-down, and #4 stretch. A warm-up, cool-down, and stretch should *always* be done!!

For fastest results, do the "mini tramp" or your walk every morning, and in addition, do an extra 15-20 minutes as many evenings as you can. Body fat almost "melts" away with *additional* aerobic activity (along with the eating plan)! Whichever you choose, while losing weight, the *minimum* number of times for your activity program must be once daily, six days each week, and the *minimum* amount of time (after beginning stage) must be 50-60 minutes. When you have reached your ideal weight, 45-55 minutes of activity four to five times a week will maintain weight very nicely for most people.

Checking Your Exercise Heart Rate

Your exercise heart rate indicates your level of exertion during your activity and is very important in making your activity *effective* as well as *safe*. To determine what your exercise heart rate should be, find your age on chart #6.1 and read the figure in the 2nd column to the right (75% of max.). Do not exceed this heart rate figure for the first *four weeks* of your activity, after which, increase intensity of activity so that your heart rate reaches 80%. These figures indicate what your *pulse* should be for one minute while you are performing your activity *after* the warm-up. You may want to divide these figures by 4 to find your pulse rate for 15 seconds rather than counting the pulse for the entire minute.

For example, for maximum benefits, a 34 year old for the first four weeks should perfom an activity fast enough to increase the heart rate to 140 beats per minute (2nd column to the right of age 34). This pulse rate for *one* minute, 140, divided by 4 = 35. So, for the first four weeks of activity for a beginning 34 year old, the exercise heart rate should be maintained at 35 beats per 15 seconds.

Two of the easiest places to locate the pulse for checking exercise heart rate are the temples and outside edge of the wrist, directly below the base of the thumb.

Place the tips of your first three fingers lightly over the pulse at the wrist or temples. Count the beats for 15 seconds and multiply by 4. This gives your heart rate for one minute. Compare with the Exercise Heart Rate Chart, #6.1.

There are several medications that affect heart rate. If you are taking any kind of medication, see your doctor and get his approval before beginning an activity program, and also ask him if the medication you are taking will affect your heart rate. If it does, use the "breathing test" instead of exercise heart rate. The breathing test is simply performing the activity with enough speed (or intensity) that there is a definite increase in breathing, but *not* to the point that you cannot carry on a conversation.

During the activity, if your pulse rate is higher than it should be as indicated on the Exercise Heart Rate Chart #6.1 or your breathing increases so much that you cannot carry on a conversation, *slow down*! Go at a slower pace and check again in a few minutes. Anytime during your activity that breathing is increased only slightly, or if your pulse rate is too low, increase intensity by increasing your speed and swinging your arms more. Check again in a few minutes.

To be effective, the activity must be at the level of exertion that produces the correct heart rate or (if on medication), produces a definite increase in breathing.

Beginning Your Fat Burning Metabolic Increasing Activity

On the following pages are step by step directions showing how to begin and how to increase your activity. Read them carefully before beginning. Remember, amounts of time are suggestions only. If you are extremely overweight, you may want to begin by doing a ten or fifteen minute activity at two different times of day. *Never proceed* to the next level until you are comfortable with the level at which you are working. Whichever you do, begin by alternating fast and slow, and always include the warm-up, EHR

Chart #6.1
RECOMMENDED HEART RATES
DURING EXERCISE

Age	80% of Max. (after 4 weeks)	75% of Max. (first 4 weeks)
20	160	150
22	158	148
24	157	147
26	155	145
28	154	144
30	152	143
32	151	142
34	150	140
36	149	140
38	147	138
40	146	137
45	143	134
50	140	131
55	137	128
60	128	120
65+	120	113

Based on resting heart rates of 72
for males and 80 for females.

(exercise heart rate) checks, cool-down, and stretches as indicated.

Following are examples of beginning levels of walking and using the mini tramp, followed by directions for increasing to each subsequent level.

Examples

Walking	Mini Tramp
1. Warm-up stroll 4 min.	1. Warm-up gentle bounce 4 min.
2. Brisk walk 5 min.	2. Jog on tramp 5 min.
3. Stroll 2 min.	3. Off tramp and walk 2 min.
4. Brisk walk 5 min.	4. Jog on tramp 5 min.
5. Check EHR	5. Check EHR
6. Stroll 2 min.	6. Off tramp and walk 2 min.
7. Brisk walk 5 min.	7. Jog on tramp 5 min.
8. Stroll 2 min.	8. Off tramp and walk 2 min.
9. Brisk walk 5 min.	9. Jog on tramp 5 min.
10. Check EHR	10. Check EHR
11. Cool down stroll 5 min	11. Cool down - gentle bounce 5 min.
12. Stretch	12. Stretch

Total Time:
30 min. + 5 min. cool-down and stretch.

Total Time:
30 min. + 5 min. cool-down and stretch.

Level 1 - Goal 30 Minutes
(Do Not Count Warm-Up)

1. Warm-up
   a. Mini tramp – gentle bounce 4 minutes.
   b. Walking – slow stroll 4 minutes.

2. Increase speed
   a. Mini tramp – jog in place 3-5 minutes.
   b. Walking – long strides, *brisk* walk 3-5 minutes.

3. Decrease speed
   a. Mini tramp – get off and walk around room 2 minutes.
   b. Walking – shorter strides, slow walk 2 minutes.

4. Alternate #2 and #3 above for a total of 25 minutes. Check EHR at *end* of the 3-5 minute increases (#2).

5. *Cool-down
   a. Mini tramp – gentle bounce 5 minutes.
   b. Walking – slow stroll 5 minutes.

6. *Stretch – (see chapter on stretching for illustrations).

* During exercise, circulation increases markedly. Without a *cool-down* and *stretch* to allow a gradual decrease in circulation, blood tends to "pool" in the blood vessels, contributing to many negative health aspects including varicose veins!

Level 2 – Goal 35 Minutes
(Do Not Count Warm-Up)

1. Warm-up
   a. Mini tramp – gentle bounce 4 minutes.
   b. Walking – slow stroll 4 minutes.

2. Increase speed to reach 75% of maximum exercise heart rate.
   a. Mini tramp – jog in place and swing arms 8-10 minutes, check EHR.

    b.   Walking – long strides, brisk walk and swing arms 8-10 minutes, check EHR.

3.   Decrease speed
    a.   Mini tramp – get off and walk around room 1-2 minutes as necessary.
    b.   Walking – shorter strides, slow walk 1-2 minutes as necessary.

4.   Alternate #2 and #3 above for a total of 30 minutes. Be sure to check EHR at the end of each increase (#2).

5.   Cool-down
    a.   Mini tramp – gentle bounce 5 minutes.
    b.   Walking – slow stroll 5 minutes.

6.   Stretch (see chapter on stretching for illustrations).

Level 3 – Goal 40 Minutes
(Do Not Count Warm-Up)

1.   Warm-up
    a.   Mini tramp – gentle bounce 4 minutes.
    b.   Walking – slow stroll 4 minutes

2.   Increase speed to reach 75% of maximum exercise heart rate.
    a.   Mini tramp – jog in place and swing arms 10-15 minutes. Check EHR.
    b.   Walking – long strides, brisk walk, swing arms, 10-15 minutes. Check EHR.

3.   Decrease speed
    a.   Mini tramp – get off and walk around room 1-2 minutes as necessary.
    b.   Walking – shorter strides, slow walk 1-2 minutes as necessary.

4.   Alternate #2 and #3 above for a total of 40 minutes. Check EHR at the end of each increase (#2).

5. Cool-down
   a. Mini tramp – gentle bounce 5 minutes.
   b. Walking – slow stroll 5 minutes

6. Stretch (see chapter on stretching for illustrations).

Level 4 – Goal 50 Minutes
(Do Not Count Warm-Up)

1. Warm-up
   a. Mini tramp – gentle bounce 4 minutes.
   b. Walking – slow stroll 4 minutes.

2. Increase speed to reach 75% of maximum exercise heart rate.
   a. Mini tramp – jog in place and swing arms 15-20 minutes. Check EHR.
   b. Walking – long strides, brisk walk, swing arms, 15-20 minutes. Check EHR.

3. Decrease speed
   a. Mini tramp – get off and walk around room 1-2 minutes as necessary.
   b. Walking – shorter strides, slow walk 1-2 minutes as necessary.

4. Alternate #2 and #3 above for a total of 50 minutes. Check EHR at the end of each increase (#2).

5. Cool-down
   a. Mini tramp – gentle bounce 5 minutes
   b. Walking – slow stroll 5 minutes.

6. Stretch (see chapter on stretching for illustrations).

Level 5 – Goal 60 Minutes
(Do Not Count Warm-Up)

1. Warm Up
    a. Mini tramp – gentle bounce 4 minutes.
    b. Walking – slow stroll 4 minutes.

2. Increase speed to reach 75% of maximum exercise heart rate.
    a. Mini tramp – jog in place and swing arms 15-20 minutes. Check EHR.
    b. Walking – long strides, brisk walk, swing arms, 15-20 minutes. Check EHR.

3. Decrease speed
    a. Mini tramp – get off and walk around room 1-2 minutes as necessary.
    b. Walking – shorter strides, slow walk 1-2 minutes as necessary.

4. Alternate #2 and #3 above for a total of 60 minutes. Check EHR at the end of each increase (#2).

5. *Cool-down
    a. Mini tramp – gentle bounce 5 minutes.
    b. Walking – slow stroll 5 minutes.

6. *Stretch (see chapter on stretching for illustrations).

You will reach your final goal in level 5. Begin to *decrease* the amount of time of the slower intervals as you comfortably can, until you are performing the entire 60 minutes of your activity within the range of 75% to 80% of your exercise heart rate. From this point on, check your heart rate at least three times throughout your activity at 20 minute intervals and adjust your speed and arm movements accordingly. Remember, your 15 second pulse rate should *never* be more than *4 beats above* or *below* your exercise heart rate range.

Activity Hints To Speed Up Weight Loss

Below is a list of helpful hints. Read them carefully and refer to them when motivation begins to wane. Make a photo copy or tear out the page and put it in a place where you will see it often.

1. Whenever you can, extend the duration of your activity sessions. Try to add ten minutes to your walking time per week until you reach your goal.

2. If you expect to be in a situation where you might eat more than usual, add one extra activity session per serving of food daily for 2 days. Do the extra activity sessions *before* you do the eating! For extra insurance, do them afterwards also.

3. Take exercise breaks. At work, go for a short walk after lunch. At home, instead of running to the kitchen when the TV commercial comes on, hop on the mini tramp or simply walk around the house until the program resumes. Food urges, unlike real hunger, will only last fifteen minutes, whether you eat or not.

4. Don't give up! You're changing your lifestyle and there is no hurry! If you miss one or two days of exercise or eat more than you intended, simply resume your program and add extra activity sessions for a day or two. Know that you are reconstructing your lifestyle and *you* are in control!

5. Beginning is half done! If you don't feel like getting started (most of us don't) promise yourself that after five minutes of the activity, if you want to quit, you may. I use this method myself, since I don't like starting, especially on cold, winter mornings. Almost 99% of the time, after I've been walking five minutes, I begin to enjoy it and choose not to quit.

6. The appetite depressant effect of the activities has helped many of the "Fat To Fit" students break the evening eating habit! When feeling the urge to snack unnecessarily in the evening, they put the mini tramp in front of the TV, hop on, and in 15-

20 minutes, the urge is gone and they've increased their activity time for the day! A bonus – you will sleep better, also!

7. Extra activity sessions while losing weight will bring quicker results. People who find time for a *second* activity session each day, even if only a 15-20 minute walk after lunch, not only lose weight faster but experience faster metabolic increases. If extra activity sessions will not fit into a busy work day schedule, try adding them to your weekends.

8. After reaching ideal weight, activity sessions usually may be cut back to 4 times weekly at 40-50 minutes each session, to maintain ideal weight and keep the basal metabolic rate increased.

9. If you think it will take too long to notice results, you are *wrong*! You will notice an increase in flexibility and mental clarity immediately, and a weight decrease the first week!

10. People who are fully trained exercisers reportedly lose only 12-15 percent of their physical condition and strength from age 21 to age 60! That statistic is enough to motivate even the most reluctant!

Questions
Increase Fat Burning and Metabolism With A Daily Walk

On the label of an aerobics video tape I just purchased, it says the program includes 12 minutes of aerobic exercise. Would this be good for me to use instead of the fast walk or mini tramp?

Most exercise video tapes are not totally aerobic exercise and therefore are not as efficient in reducing body fat. Having 12 minutes of "aerobic" exercise is not an accurate statement. To be "aerobic," the *minimum* amount of time must be 25-30 minutes.

Aerobic exercise is a specific for reducing body fat by increasing fat burning and metabolism – increases which continue for as long as fifteen hours *after* the activity is over! However, to be aerobic, an activity must include three essential aspects: 1) intensity to elevate heart rate to 70-80 percent of maximum (see Exercise Heart Rate Chart), 2) a minimum duration of 25-30 minutes, and 3) an increase in maximum oxygen uptake.

You will use calories when you do exercises that are not aerobic, but the fat burning effect and the metabolic increases are left to aerobic activities.

I've tried aerobics classes, but I get very tired and I cannot keep up. In addition, I am so sore the next day I can hardly move! I like the mini trampoline, but is it as good for reducing body fat?

Better! You set your own pace, based on your heart rate, and get a *totally* aerobic exercise that will be much more efficient at reducing body fat. "No pain, no gain," is definitely not the case!

Even better, when you are on and off the tramp (as recommended) you are doing "interval" aerobics. Research has shown that "interval" aerobics reduces body fat even quicker and also has an edge on improving cardio-vascular functions.

If you are feeling tired and sore after every class, you are overworking, which is counterproductive! If aerobic exercise is performed correctly there will be a noticeable physical and mental improvement upon the completion of the exercise. There are only two things that will prevent this: 1) if you are overworking during the exercise beyond your exercise heart rate, or 2) if your normal physical state is below par from lack of sleep, illness, etc.

Why is it that the first 15 or 20 minutes of my activity seem the hardest? After that, the rest of the hour is fine!

This is perfectly normal, and occurs in most people. Allowing an adequate time for warm-up will alleviate this somewhat. The first 15 minutes usually seem a little more difficult, but about 20 minutes into the activity your body will seem to "shift gears" and by the time you finish, you'll feel even better than before you began.

I've just started using the mini trampoline this week, and since I want to get results as quickly as possible, I am forcing myself to stay on as long as I can. I am only up to 15 minutes and even this makes me very tired. When will it get better? I can't imagine doing an hour!

Your 15 minutes non-stop on the mini tramp is too much for a non-exercising beginner! What you are doing is tiring yourself out and getting nowhere. At only 15 minutes, you are not getting into the fat burning or the metabolic increases at all, therefore your efforts are practically wasted!

If you do the interval – on and off the mini tramp as suggested, you will not get tired and you will be able to go for a longer period of time to get beyond the critical 20 minute point. It is only after the first 20 minutes that your body begins burning fat and you get the metabolic increases. At 15 minutes non-stop you're not getting the benefits, you are only getting *tired*!

Go back and read the directions for beginning your activity and make sure you do the intervals – on and off the mini tramp as suggested, and your results *and* energy will be markedly improved.

I have been fast-walking for quite a while. I don't seem to be working as hard as I did in the beginning. Is this to be expected?

The first thing you need to do is check your EHR (exercise heart rate). Some people get lax and stop checking EHR soon after they become accustomed to their activity. This is a mistake! You should continue to check EHR at least twice during each activity to make sure you are within your target heart rate zone. If you are walking for one full hour and are not maintaining your EHR you will not get the benefits of the activity. To get the fat reduction and the metabolic increases, you *must* maintain your EHR!

The following is a typical example. Betty was fast walking and checked her EHR faithfully for about six weeks. At that time she figured that her walking would always increase her heart rate to her target zone and she stopped checking. Six weeks later, she stopped losing weight and was totally confused as to why. She was reminded to check her EHR, which she did, and was surprised to find that it was much lower than it should have been. Therefore, her walking was no longer aerobic.

Both cardio-vascular health and endurance improve as you continue your activity. This is good but it also means that from time to time you must increase your intensity and work a little harder as indicated by your EHR. Otherwise your activity will not be productive. If you discontinue checking your EHR you won't know when to increase intensity.

Betty found another route to walk that included some hills, and once again she began maintaining her EHR, and she also began losing weight again.

For best results, continue to check EHR at least *twice* during each session, to make sure your activity is effective and will give you the results you want.

With my schedule, I cannot possibly find one full hour in the morning or evening for my activity. Any suggestions?

I don't know what your schedule is like, but here are some daily alternatives:

1. 30 minutes - AM (get up 30 minutes earlier)
    20-30 minutes - lunchtime and/or
    30 minutes - PM

2. Park 30 minutes from your work and walk AM and PM. Also walk for a few minutes after lunch, if possible.

3. Take a mini trampoline to work and try to get 2 or 3 sessions of 25 minutes a day. It can be propped up against a wall when not in use. I used to take mine to work and jogged 30 minutes at lunch and 40 minutes immediately after work before leaving for home.

*   One hour on Saturday and again on Sunday in addition to one of these three daily will be a big help.

If my EHR is 36 when I first begin, should I try to increase it after I've been exercising a few months?

No! As stated previously, your cardio-vascular health improves and after a few months you'll have to work a little harder to reach the 36, but *never* go above the number indicated on the Exercise Heart Rate Chart.

Can I lose weight without doing the activity?

No. You would have to cut back caloric intake which would slow the metabolism and then your problems would be worse.

The body tends to try to maintain "status quo." Increasing the metabolism is difficult if not impossible without using both the dietary and activity approaches. People who have tried one without the other invariably fail!

I have "cellulite" as well as excess fat on my thighs and have been doing leg exercises for six months, but my legs still don't look any better. What can I do?

"Cellulite" is fat which causes "dimpling" as it pushes up between connective tissue under the skin. Women's connective tissue is not as strong as men's, therefore women usually have more problems with cellulite. Since cellulite is fat, reducing body fat will also reduce cellulite.

Leg exercises will not get rid of cellulite! What is needed is aerobic activity to reduce body fat, which includes cellulite on hips, stomach, thighs, or wherever the fat happens to be.

Many people will do a hundred or more abdominal exercises every day in a very heroic attempt to "flatten" this area. While these exercises help to strengthen and firm the abdominal muscles, the layer of fat which is situated on *top* of these muscles will remain, causing the abdominal area to protrude unless some type of aerobic activity is included.

Are there benefits other than weight loss in doing the activity?

Absolutely! The following is a *partial* list of some of the proven and documented benefits of regular aerobic activity:

1. Increased mental and physical energy accompanied by an elevation in mood.
2. Resting heart rate decreased.
3. Normal heart rate decreased throughout daily activities.
4. Hypertensive people show a decrease in blood pressure.
5. Oxygen uptake increased with subsequent increases to muscles and skin.
6. Increased oxygen and circulation. (Keeps skin younger looking, helps prevent and diminish wrinkles.)
7. Causes firming of muscles and decrease in fat.
8. Increased strength of tendons, ligaments and muscles.
9. Increased density and strength of bones.
10. Helps prevent osteoporosis.
11. Helps control diabetes.
12. Strengthens and enhances health of heart, lungs and circulatory system.
13. Decreased triglycerides and cholesterol.
14. Decreased fatigue, increased energy levels.
15. Increased fat utilization and metabolism even at rest.
16. Decreased constipation.
17. Relieves stress.
18. Contributes to deeper more restful sleep.
19. Decreased appetite.
20. Increased oxygen to brain (contributes to mental alertness).

7

STRETCHING MOVEMENTS

It is very important to cool down and stretch at the *end* of each activity. The following illustrations will stretch and add flexibility to all the major muscle groups of the body. It is a brief stretching program, but nevertheless a very important part of your activity.

Take your time and do the stretches as if you were moving in slow motion. Avoid fast or "jerky" movements. Never "bounce," but slowly reach the fullest comfortable position and hold for a slow count of twelve. Move slowly from one position to the next, and modify any move so that you feel a good stretch. Never force your muscles into a move and never increase a stretch to the point of discomfort or pain.

You'll be amazed at your increased flexibility which will help you move about in your day to day activities with more agility. If you are presently experiencing any body stiffness, you'll notice a dramatic improvement.

#1
WING SPREAD
(pectoral, shoulder and upper back muscles)

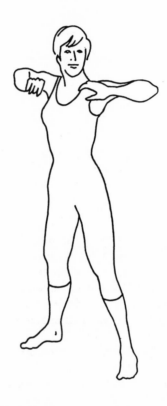

1. Stand with feet approximately 12 inches apart with elbows straight out from shoulders.

2. Push elbows slowly back as far as is comfortable and hold for a slow count of 12.

3. Return to starting position.

#2
SIDE STRETCH
(trunk, arm and neck muscles)

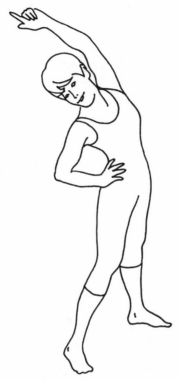

1. Stand erect, with both hands overhead, interlocked and with palms toward ceiling.

2. Lean to right side, making sure left arm is beside left ear, right hand on waist, making sure there is no back discomfort. Hold for slow count of 12.

3. Move slowly to left side repeating move, with right arm beside right ear and left hand on waist. Hold for slow count of 12.

4. Stretch both arms directly overhead at end of move.

#3
BACK LEG WALL STRETCH
(calf and hamstring muscles)

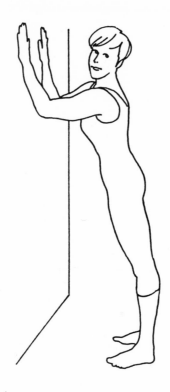

1. Stand approximately 3 feet from a wall with feet together.

2. Put hands on wall.

3. Keeping heels on floor lean into wall, bend elbows and touch head to wall.

4. Keep back in straight line with legs.

5. Hold for slow count of 12.

#4
KNEE BEND
(thigh and trunk muscles)

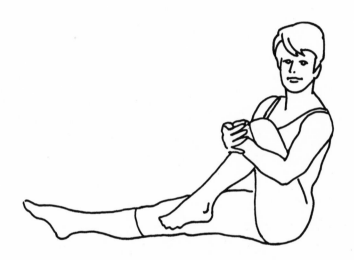

1. Seated on floor, legs extended straight ahead, pull left leg as close to chest as possible, keeping back straight.

2. Hold for slow count of 12.

3. Repeat with right leg.

#5
TOE TOUCH
(lower back, hamstring, and thigh muscles)

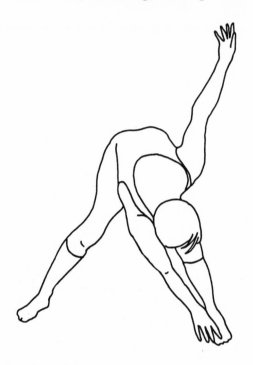

1. Stand erect, arms spread at sides, shoulder height, feet 16-18 inches apart.

2. Bend knees slightly, slowly twist trunk and touch right hand to left foot.

3. Hold for a slow count of 12.

4. Repeat with left hand to right foot.

#6
INNER THIGH STRETCH
(inner thigh, hip muscles)

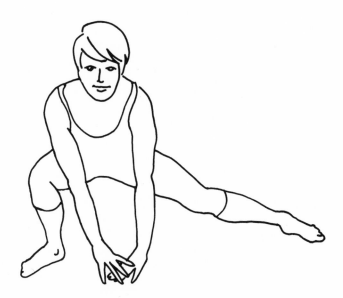

1. Bend knees slightly and put hands in front of feet on floor.

2. Slide left foot to left side with foot <u>flat</u> on floor and left leg straight out from left side.

3. Keep right knee directly over right toes, hands on floor directly in front to support your body.

4. Hold for slow count of 12.

5. Repeat to right, keeping right foot flat on floor and keeping left knee directly over left foot.

#7
OVERHEAD BODY STRETCH
(shoulder, arm, back, chest, leg muscles)

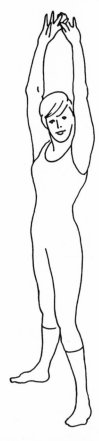

1. With feet wide apart, stretch arms overhead.

2. Reach as high as possible. Hold for a slow 12 count.

3. Drop arms to sides, let head roll easily to front, relax shoulders. Hold for a slow count of 12.

4. Repeat.

Questions
Stretching Movements

Is it absolutely necessary to do the stretches after every activity, even in the beginning?

Yes! They will help you cool down and will also add to your flexibility.

There are two or three other stretching moves I learned in an exercise class that I would like to add to the suggested stretches. Would there be a problem with adding these?

Not at all as long as you follow the basic guidelines of moving slowly, holding the stretch and avoiding jerky or bouncing moves.

Stretch #5, the Toe Touch, gives me some problems. I cannot touch my toes, and wonder if the stretch will be effective this way.

Yes, it will be effective. Any move illustrated must be modified to suit your present beginning flexibility. Always proceed in a move only to the point that will stretch muscles. You should never force muscles or feel any pain. Take each movement just to the point of a good stretch – never pain, and never force your body into the full position.

The hamstring muscles in the backs of the legs are usually "tight" in people who have never used stretching exercises or have not used them on a regular basis, but will improve dramatically if you perform these exercises on a daily basis.

The knee bend, #4 is difficult for me to do because of my large abdomen. Should I continue this stretch?

Yes, continue the stretch, but modify your movement so that you are comfortable with it and feel a stretch in the thigh muscles in the front of the upper leg.

I feel the Side Stretch, #2 in my back. Am I doing something wrong?

Yes. Make sure your upper arm is always beside your ear. If this doesn't help, stand with your right side about 2 feet from a wall. Put your right hand on the wall for support and lean over to the wall with your left arm beside your left ear, touching your left hand to the wall and hold for a slow 12 count. Repeat on the other side.

When doing the Inner Thigh Stretch, #6, why is it necessary to have your bent knee directly over your toes?

To prevent stress on the knee joint. When your flexibility increases to the point that the inner thigh does not seem to be stretched adequately in this position, move the straight leg out farther from the body – *never* bend knee farther!

Why is it necessary to keep the foot of the straight leg flat on the floor when doing #6, Inner Thigh Stretch?

Keeping the foot flat avoids stress on knee joints. When the foot is allowed to roll on the side, the knee joint is stressed.

The Back Leg Wall Stretch, #3, causes back discomfort. Am I performing it incorrectly?

Back discomfort will occur if you allow your pelvis to "dip" into the wall you're facing, causing the back to curve in rather than keeping it straight. Try performing the exercise where there is a mirror that you can use to see if your back is in a straight line as illustrated.

I have been doing the stretching exercises for about two months and I can feel a big difference in ease of movement, especially when I've been sitting for a period of time and then get up. Also, my back does not hurt as much. Could I safely do these stretches more often?

Please do! You might want to perform each one *twice* instead of once, if you like. You are absolutely right – flexibility increases make all movements easier! Do make sure you never stretch without first warming your muscles with activity.

8

THE FAT TO FIT WEIGHT LOSS PLAN

The Eating Plan

The "Fat to Fit Weight Loss Plan" is very thorough in its approach. The eating plan itself, while simple in design, allows for a natural progression through the following three components: 1) *Daily Menus* (a structured beginning in which menus are planned for you), 2) *Overview* (guidelines to assist you in choosing your own foods and menus) and 3) *Quick Weight Loss* (to reverse the effects of an occasional overindulgence). Each provides very pleasurable eating that increases metabolism and fat burning processes to produce weight loss that is natural and permanent without calorie restriction.

For best results it is recommended that you begin with the *Daily Menus* for the first four weeks, then follow the *Overview* to assist in planning your own menus for subsequent weeks, and reserve the *Quick Weight Loss* for an "emergency repair kit" following an occasional overindulgence.

In following the plan, eating habits are changed so that food is used to nourish the body rather than fatten it. This produces very noticeable health and energy improvements along with weight control.

94

Not a diet, it is designed so that no food is eliminated and eating is very pleasurable as nature intended. Anything less is doomed to failure, a very difficult concept for overweight people to grasp. Time after time, these people have been led to believe their enjoyment of eating has caused their problems and therefore they must live in a constant state of hunger and eat tasteless diet foods to lose weight. These are the ideas that have perpetuated all the no-win diet situations.

Hard as it is to believe, making sure you are eating foods you enjoy will help to insure your success. It is important that your menus include foods you would rate, on a scale of 1-10, no lower than a 6 or 7. Enjoying the foods you eat is extremely important in helping you make permanent changes in your eating habits.

The goal of the eating plan is to change "fat" eating habits, which does not necessarily mean "over-eating" habits. As we know, most overweight people are already eating less than their thin friends. Changing "fat" eating habits, means putting into practice the unique combination of scientifically proven principles to increase metabolism so that the body uses food for energy rather than fat production.

Following these principles, more of your food is eaten earlier in the day and is divided into three meals and three snacks (six smaller feedings). Fiber and complex carbohydrate intake is high, protein is moderate, with fats and sugars low. Supplements as listed are your option, but are highly recommended.

The step by step directions for getting started are as simple, brief and thorough as possible, to avoid confusion. Having been an avid reader of diet books for many years, the thing that I found most frustrating was having to "wade" through 16 pages of information to find out what to have for breakfast! Some books would require you to refer to 6 or 7 different lists or "exchanges" that seemed to require a CPA to figure out. This eating plan is simple to follow, but the first week or two will require extra time and effort, not because of the difficulty of the eating plan, but because you're breaking a habit – your old eating habit. Breaking a habit, no matter what the habit is, takes time, patience, and a concerted effort. Be patient with yourself and remember that a "mistake" in reality, is a "learning situation" – accept it as such and let it be part of your progress!

Four Weekly Menus

You will be given planned menus for the first four weeks. By week five you may use guidelines to help you design your own menus based on your food preferences and choices. The first week's menu allows you many delicious foods, but the design is more strict than later weeks simply to facilitate the learning that must occur in order for you to make appropriate changes in your eating habits. It is more structured with fewer choices so that you can begin with as little confusion as possible. Weeks two through four are designed much like a restaurant menu with two to three choices for each meal and snack every day, providing more choices and options. After these four weeks you will plan your own menu with the option of using previous menus, the suggested meals and snacks, or your own favorite foods, including desserts, if you wish. In this respect, there is a planned progression.

The menus on the following pages are provided for the first 4 weeks for several important purposes.

First, they give you examples to guide you in subsequent weeks when planning your own menu. It is very important that you try the foods before you decide whether or not you like them. If you find there is a food you don't like, refer to the "Meals and Snacks Suggestions" and substitute a food you like. Be sure to note the substitution you make on your Eating Plan. Never substitute a P/F meal or snack for one that is *not* P/F! (P/F – a protein in which the fat content is fairly high.)

Second, the menus introduce you to some of the recipes that otherwise you may not try, and I can understand your reluctance. As a former fat person, I must have gone through at least a hundred or more low calorie recipes, none of which could be tolerated well enough to get past my nose! I decided it was time to take to the kitchen and try my hand at putting together some really good tasting, non-fattening recipes. I must admit that there were a lot even "Rebel" (our German Shepherd) would not eat, but there were also some that turned out top notch! You're in for a real gourmet treat when you make the cheese cake that tastes just like (or even better than) the "real McCoy," *without* all the fat and sugar! The Acidophilus Shake is a favorite and most popular item at the Snack Bar in our fitness club, as well as with the "Fat To Fit" students.

You won't believe that this thick and creamy "milkshake" has *no* fat, *no* sugar and yet delivers 30 grams of protein!

Third, for people who are busy and don't like to plan menus, the first four weeks are already planned for you and may be used as often as you like. Just one word of caution – don't neglect variety in your choice of foods! There are many choices you can make.

Fourth, having the first four weeks of menus planned for you allows you to begin your program with as little effort as possible. Be sure to use each week's menu to compile your grocery list.

Preparing Yourself To Begin

Before you begin your weight loss program, it is essential that you read "Weight Loss Special Notes" on the following pages. There is much information you need to know about different food choices listed on your menus – which cereals are sugar-free, which cheeses are low-fat, which beverages are best to drink, etc.

Also, plan a time when it will be most convenient for you to do your activity. On your first day, be sure to fill in your beginning weight and measurements on your "Master Success Record."

One word of caution – although I have worked with people well over 300 pounds, it is always best to check with your doctor before beginning the suggested activity, or any activity. This is especially true if you are severely overweight or if you have any medical problems. You will likely receive your doctor's blessing, but it is best to be sure.

The questions appearing at the end of this chapter will clarify some important points. Be sure to read them carefully.

Weight Loss Special Notes

The following are special notes, concise and in list form, to be used as a quick reference for essential information needed throughout your weight loss program. Be sure to read thoroughly and become familiar with them before beginning your first week.

1. Coffee or teas, if desired, in moderation, 3-4 cups daily. Any other sugar-free beverage in moderation. Fruit juices should be omitted or mixed half and half with water (2 oz. juice with 2 oz. water) in the morning only.

2. Use fat-free powdered milk as a powdered "creamer" in coffee or tea, if desired – 1 tsp./serving.

3. Diet soda – choose those that are *sodium, caffeine* and *sugar-free*. It is best to limit to one per day or *less*, so that the habit of drinking water is encouraged.

4. Until you reach your weight goal, it is best to plan menus *one week* in advance and use the menu plan for your grocery shopping list.

5. Sweetener – "Equal," or "Sweet'n Low," or any other brand. Use as desired.

6. NEVER skip meals or snacks! Eat only part of a meal or snack if you are not hungry. Modify, *do not omit*!

7. Use greens other than lettuce to add variety to salads – kale, endive, raw sprouts, raw spinach, etc.

8. Begin eating dinner at least 4-5 hours before bedtime.

9. All meats are to be broiled, steamed, or baked – no breading or frying. Remove all visible fat and remove skin from turkey, chicken or other poultry.

10. Use Morton's Lite Salt, Mrs. Dash, or other salt substitutes or herb mixtures in place of regular salt if you are a "big salt" eater.

11. Cold cereals, if desired, should be Kellogg's Nutri Grain (corn, nuggets, or wheat), Grape Nuts (*not* Grape Nut Flakes), Shredded Wheat, Puffed Rice, Sun Flakes, or Nabisco's Shredded Wheat 'N' Bran.

12. Use "Butter Buds" powder straight from packet or mix with water, or use a diet margarine.

13. Be CREATIVE!! If "addicted" to potato chips or a "crunchy" snack, try munching on 1/3 cup dry Kellogg's Nutri Grain cereal flakes – plain or lightly tossed with 1 tsp. of Butter Buds powder. (Take with you in a plastic zip-top baggie). Slice your carrot snacks in bite-sized pieces and munch throughout snack time rather than all at one time. Snacks may be set out in a convenient place (on your desk at work) and munched a little at a time or eaten all at one time, whichever you prefer.

14. DRINK WATER!! Fat loss may be hampered if the body does not get enough water in order to perform the many necessary chemical processes. Put it in a thermos and sip throughout the day if this is a problem for you. Start with 1 quart a day and work up to a minimum of 2 quarts a day. Fluid retention is often a result of not drinking enough water. The body tends to "hold onto" the water it has to fulfill its needs, "knowing" there's not much water coming in.

15. If you "slip," walk or jog on a mini tramp an extra session before retiring for the evening and try to get another *extra* activity session in the next day. Or, follow the "Quick Weight Loss Plan" for one or two days. (See "Quick Weight Loss Plan," chapter 9.)

16. Keep a non-perishable "emergency snack" in your car or at work if you anticipate ever having to miss a snack.

17. Avoid "creamed" soups, and have "broth" soups instead. Homemade is best (see recipe) followed by Lipton's "Lite" cup of soup, but do watch the sodium content!

18. If you are going out for dinner or to a party, *always* eat a small baked potato or 1/2 bagel with light cream cheese *before leaving home*, or on the way to the event, so you do not arrive hungry!

19. Raw vegetables are permitted in unlimited amounts in addition to regular snacks, anytime you feel hungry.

20. Limit beef to twice weekly, pork to once in two weeks and make it *lean*. Best meats to have most frequently: 1) skinless turkey and chicken (especially the breast), 2) fish, 3) seafood (limit crabmeat, shrimp and oysters to 4 oz. once or twice weekly if you have a cholesterol problem). All should be baked, broiled or steamed without breading.

21. If your family demands large evening meals every evening, and you prefer to eat with them, follow these guidelines: a) *Always* have an "appetizer" right before dinner or while fixing dinner! Choose *one* of the following for appetizer:
    • 1/2 Acidophilus Shake (drink other half with or after meal for a PM snack).
    • 1 cup (broth only) soup plus 1 diet slice whole wheat bread.
    • 1/2 slice low-fat cheese on 1 diet slice whole wheat bread.
    • 1 diet slice whole wheat bread with 2 tsp. peanut butter.
    • tossed salad with dressing (see recipe).
    b) Your dinner should be *child*-sized portions *only*! c) Arrange food from family's dinner on a microwave dish, with lid, and eat your dinner-sized portions for lunch the next day. This is a great time-saver and an extremely convenient way to pack lunches! d) No regular dessert foods for the first 4-6 weeks.
    Note: For the individual whose family eats high fat foods such as ham, pizza, hamburgers, hot dogs, etc. for most evening meals, it would be best to have only the veggies and limit these high fat foods to one serving of 1/2-1 oz.

22. Low-fat cheese slices – *Country Singles, Nu Form, or Lite 'N Lively*. These taste just like American Cheese, but fat content is 1 1/2 grams per slice as compared to American Cheese at 7-9 grams per slice. But don't get carried away because sodium content is very high!

23. You may increase serving sizes of foods both at *breakfast* and *lunch*, if your appetite is not satisfied with suggested

amounts. Eat only until satisfied – *never* eat until you are too full! Make sure you are never hungry, but never stuffed! Adjust portions of food accordingly.

24. Anytime you are feeling tired for *no apparent reason*, and/or you are experiencing *real* hunger in the evenings, you should increase complex carbohydrate intake at the afternoon snack. (Complex carbohydrates: 1) all vegetables, 2) any food made from grains – cereals, breads, pop corn, etc.) A bagel, baked potato, pop corn, etc. make good afternoon snacks. If this does not end evening hunger, increase the amount of food for lunch in addition to afternoon snack, or have 2 afternoon snacks – raw veggies for early afternoon and a regular snack for late afternoon.

25. When eating out late or unexpectedly, choose a restaurant with a soup and salad bar and eat a large salad with dressing as described in "recipes." If there is no salad bar, order 2 salads (eat the first as an appetizer, the second with meal) plus a small serving of a cooked veggie, 3-4 oz. *broiled* fish or chicken and "doggie bag" any "left-overs" for the next day's lunch!

26. Do not use *instant* hot cereals. Use regular oatmeal (see recipe – "Hot Cereal") or cook regular cereal ahead of time and re-heat as needed in double boiler or microwave.

27. Men may add *daily* 2 more grain servings (cereals, bread, crackers, etc.), plus an additional 2 oz. of meat, fish, poultry or seafood per serving.

28. Bread – use whole wheat diet or extra thin slices for lunch, dinner and PM snacks. Use regular whole grain breads for breakfast and afternoon snacks.

29. You *must* do your Activity Plan *every* day until you reach your weight goal.

30. Read and re-read "Weight Loss Special Notes" *every* day until

you are very familiar with them. Then re-read once or twice weekly until you reach your weight goal.

31. Choose the right vegetables for each meal. At lunch you may have any vegetable you want. At dinner, however, choose light vegetables such as kale, brussels sprouts, broccoli, green beans, asparagus, onions, carrots, etc. You may also have "seed type" vegetables such as corn, rice, lima beans, and potatoes but only in very small amounts.

Note: If you choose *NOT* to use amino acid supplements, you may substitute *ONE* of the following wherever "Amino Acids" appear on menus:
    1) 3 egg whites, cooked
    2) 2/3 cup fat-free yogurt
    3) 2/3 cup low-fat cottage cheese
    4) 1/2 can plain white tuna (packed in water)

Master Success Record

Enter your weight and measurements on the beginning day of your program, and again at the end of each week. Be sure to measure accurately with a *snug*, not *tight* measuring tape! Weigh yourself first thing in the morning without clothes. Weigh and measure once a week *only!*

Master Success Record

Weight

Beginning Weight Day 1 _____
Weight Day 8 _____   _____ Lost Week 1
Weight Day 15 _____   _____ Lost Week 2
Weight Day 22 _____   _____ Lost Week 3
Weight Day 29 _____   _____ Lost Week 4

Inches – Chest

Beginning Day 1 _____
Day 8 _____   _____ Lost Week 1
Day 15 _____   _____ Lost Week 2
Day 22 _____   _____ Lost Week 3
Day 29 _____   _____ Lost Week 4

Waist

Beginning Day 1 _____
Day 8 _____   _____ Lost Week 1
Day 15 _____   _____ Lost Week 2
Day 22 _____   _____ Lost Week 3
Day 29 _____   _____ Lost Week 4

Hips

Beginning Day 1 _____
Day 8 _____   _____ Lost Week 1
Day 15 _____   _____ Lost Week 2
Day 22 _____   _____ Lost Week 3
Day 29 _____   _____ Lost Week 4

Upper Right and Left Thigh

Beginning Day 1 R_____ L_____
Day 8 R_____ L_____   _____ Lost Week 1
Day 15 R_____ L_____   _____ Lost Week 2
Day 22 R_____ L_____   _____ Lost Week 3
Day 29 R_____ L_____   _____ Lost Week 4

Totals - Four Weeks

_____ Pounds Lost   _____ Inches Lost

Weekly Success Record

Week #1
Weight

Beginning weight – Day 1 ___   Total lost this week ___
Today's weight – Day 8   ___   Total lost to date   ___

* Always weigh yourself first thing in the morning without
   clothes or shoes.

Measurements

Beginning – Day 1	Day 8	Total lost
chest ___	chest ___	___
waist ___	waist ___	___
upper rt. thigh ___	upper rt. thigh ___	___
upper lt. thigh ___	upper lt. thigh ___	___
hips ___	hips ___	___

* Inches lost will be more dramatic than pounds lost when you're
   losing body fat. One pound of fat takes up approximately five
   times the space of one pound of lean!

Activity

Goal – 30 minutes by day 7

Day 1 – Total Time ___   Day 7 – Total Time ___

Water

Day 1 – drank ——— cups   Day 2 – drank ——— cups

Day 3 – drank ——— cups   Day 4 – drank ——— cups

Day 5 – drank ——— cups   Day 6 – drank ——— cups

Day 7 – drank ——— cups

Energy Level
(Check One)

Day 1 ___ Good ___ Not Good ___ Improving ___ Not Improving

Day 2 ___ Good ___ Not Good ___ Improving ___ Not Improving

Day 3 ___ Good ___ Not Good ___ Improving ___ Not Improving

Day 4 ___ Good ___ Not Good ___ Improving ___ Not Improving

Day 5 ___ Good ___ Not Good ___ Improving ___ Not Improving

Day 6 ___ Good ___ Not Good ___ Improving ___ Not Improving

Day 7 ___ Good ___ Not Good ___ Improving ___ Not Improving

* Anytime you are feeling tired for no apparent reason, and/or you are experiencing real hunger in the evenings, you should *increase* complex carbohydrates. First, increase afternoon snacks – whole grain bagel, popcorn, 1/2-1 sandwich on whole grain bread, etc. If tiredness or evening hunger persists, increase food intake at lunch in addition.

Week 1

I. Beginning Weight and Measurements

Weigh yourself in the morning, nude, and record weight on both your Master Success Record, and Weekly Success Record. After recording weight, measure with a snug, not tight, measuring tape and record as indicated on Master Success Record and Weekly Success Record.

II. Activity Plan

Read over Activity Plans for day #1. Compute and record in a convenient place, your 15 second exercise heart rate (EHR). You may begin your Activity either on the same day or before you begin your Eating Plan. Be sure to read chapter on stretching.

III. Eating Plan

A. Read over first week's menu and list groceries you must get.

B. Check ingredients for the following recipes that you will need this week and add to grocery list:
   1. Acidophilus Shake
   2. Hot Cereal
   3. Jello
   4. Fudgesicles
   5. Whipped Cream Cheese
   6. Onion Dip
   7. Strawberry Jelly
   8. Cheese Cake (optional)

C. Make any of the recipes that you can ahead of time.

D. The word "meat" on menus also includes poultry, fish and seafood.

E. Read "Weight Loss Special Notes" carefully before beginning week #1.

**Day 1 – Monday

MENU	ACTIVITY

MENU

BREAKFAST
1/2 English Muffin w/ 1 tsp. margarine
*hot cereal (amount desired)
4 amino acid tablets

A.M. SNACK
1 small piece fresh raw fruit

LUNCH
lean meat - 4-6 oz.
small baked potato w/ 1 tsp. margarine or 1 tbsp. sour cream
*tossed salad or cooked veggie
or
4-6 oz. lean meat in sandwich with thin sliced whole grain bread, lettuce, tomato (2 tbsp. *mayo if desired) plus salad w/ *dressing or 1 cup soup

AFTERNOON SNACK
raw veggies w/ 1/2 cup *onion dip

DINNER
*Acidophilus Shake (1/2 before dinner as appetizer)
2 oz. lean meat
1/2 cup green beans *or* broccoli (meat and veggies optional)

EVENING SNACK
*jello, unlimited
or
raw veggies

How much water today? _____
*   See Recipes
**   See "Weight Loss Special Notes" *before* beginning Week I Eating Plan.

ACTIVITY
1) Walking or 2) Mini Tramp

1) Walking
1. Warm up stroll - 4 min.
2. Alternate brisk walk and stroll:
   - Brisk walk - 3 min.
   - Stroll - 2 min.
   - Brisk walk - 3 min.
   - Check EHR
   - Stroll - 2 min.
   - Brisk walk - 3 min.
   - Check EHR
   - Stroll - 2 min.
   - Brisk walk - 3 min.
3. Cool down stroll 5 min.
4. Stretch (see illustrations)

Total time - 22 min.
(Do Not Count Cool Down)

2) Mini Tramp
1. Warm up gentle bounce - 4 min.
2. Alternate on and off tramp:
   - Jog in place - 3 min.
   - Walk around room - 2 min.
   - Jog in place - 3 min.
   - Check EHR
   - Walk around room - 2 min.
   - Jog in place - 3 min.
   - Check EHR
   - Walk around room - 2 min.
   - Jog in place - 3 min.
3. Cool down gentle bounce - 5 min.
4. Stretch

Total time - 22 min.
(Do Not Count Cool Down)

How Did You Do?
1) Goal - 22 min.
2) Actual Time _____
3) Goal Reached?   Yes   No
4) EHR? High Low Just Right

Day 2 – Tuesday

MENU	ACTIVITY

ACTIVITY
1) Walking or 2) Mini Tramp

BREAKFAST
1/2 cup fat-free milk
1/2 cup sugar-free cereal and
Equal to sweeten (#11 "Weight
Loss Special Notes")
1 whole grain toast with
1 melted low-fat cheese slice

1) Walking
1. Warm up stroll - 4 min.
2. Alternate brisk walk and
   stroll:
   • Brisk walk - 3 min.
   • Stroll - 2 min.
   • Brisk walk - 3 min.
   • Check EHR
   • Stroll - 2 min.
   • Brisk walk - 3 min.
   • Check EHR
   • Stroll - 2 min.
   • Brisk walk - 3 min.

A.M. SNACK
*1/2 cup fat-free yogurt or
cottage cheese with fruit
or
1 small piece fresh raw fruit

3. Cool down stroll 5 min.
4. Stretch (see illustrations)

Total time - 22 min.
(Do Not Count Cool Down)

LUNCH P/F
lean meat (4-6 oz.) on sandwich
w/ thin sliced WW bread,
lettuce, tomato (1 tbsp. *mayo,
optional)
1 large salt-free pretzel
   (optional)
1 cup soup

2) Mini Tramp
1. Warm up gentle bounce - 4
   min.
2. Alternate on and off tramp:
   • Jog in place - 3 min.
   • Walk around room - 2 min.
   • Jog in place - 3 min.
   • Check EHR
   • Walk around room - 2 min.
   • Jog in place - 3 min.
   • Check EHR
   • Walk around room - 2 min.
   • Jog in place - 3 min.

AFTERNOON SNACK
3 cups fat-free popcorn, sprinkle
w/ Butter Buds powder or 1
tbsp. Parmesan cheese

DINNER
*Acidophilus Shake (1/2 before
dinner as appetizer)
2-4 oz. turkey or chicken breast
1/4 cup rice or 1/2 small potato
1/2 cup kale, green beans, or
asparagus

3. Cool down gentle bounce - 5
   min.
4. Stretch (see illustrations)
   Total time - 22 min.
(Do Not Count Cool Down)

EVENING SNACK
*2 fudgesicles

How much water today? _____

*   See Recipes

How Did You Do?
1) Goal - 22 min.
2) Actual Time _____
3) Goal Reached?   Yes   No
4) EHR? High Low Just Right

Day 3 – Wednesday

MENU	ACTIVITY

ACTIVITY
1) Walking or 2) Mini Tramp

MENU

BREAKFAST
3 eggs (remove 2 yolks)
scrambled in non-stick pan
2 WW toast w/ 1 tsp. margarine
on each
2 pieces Canadian bacon
(optional)
or
Have Monday's breakfast

1) Walking
1. Warm up stroll - 4 min.
2. Alternate brisk walk and
   stroll:
   • Brisk walk - 3 min.
   • Stroll - 2 min.
   • Brisk walk - 3 min.
   • Check EHR
   • Stroll - 2 min.
   • Brisk walk - 3 min.
   • Check EHR
   • Stroll - 2 min.
   • Brisk walk - 3 min.
3. Cool down stroll 5 min.
4. Stretch (see illustrations)

A.M. SNACK
1 small piece fresh raw fruit

Total time - 22 min.
(Do Not Count Cool Down)

LUNCH P/F
*turkey or chicken salad
   (2/3 cup)
2 wasa bread, rice cakes or
3 WW crackers
1 cup soup (optional)

2) Mini Tramp
1. Warm up gentle bounce - 4 min.
2. Alternate on and off tramp:
   • Jog in place - 3 min.
   • Walk around room - 2 min.
   • Jog in place - 3 min.
   • Check EHR
   • Walk around room - 2 min.
   • Jog in place - 3 min.
   • Check EHR
   • Walk around room - 2 min.
   • Jog in place - 3 min.
3. Cool down gentle bounce - 5 min.
4. Stretch (see illustrations)

AFTERNOON SNACK
small baked potato with 1 slice
low-fat cheese melted on top
or
1/2 whole grain bagel w/ 2 tsp.
peanut butter

DINNER
*Acidophilus Shake (1/2 before
dinner as appetizer)
2 oz. lean meat
1/2 cup cooked or raw veggies
(meat, veggies optional)

Total time - 22 min.
(Do Not Count Cool Down)

EVENING SNACK
2 cups fat-free popcorn
or
raw veggies

How much water today? _____

*   See Recipes

How Did You Do?
1) Goal - 22 min.
2) Actual Time _____
3) Goal Reached?   Yes   No
4) EHR? High Low Just Right

Day 4 – Thursday

MENU	ACTIVITY

ACTIVITY

1) Walking or 2) Mini Tramp

MENU

BREAKFAST

1 large raisin bagel - split and toast, spread w/ 2 tbsp. Philadelphia Light Cream Cheese and sprinkle w/ 1 Equal, if desired
4 amino acid tablets

1) Walking

1. Warm up stroll - 4 min.
2. Alternate brisk walk and stroll:
   - Brisk walk - 4 min.
   - Stroll - 2 min.
   - Brisk walk - 4 min.
   - Check EHR
   - Stroll - 2 min.
   - Brisk walk - 4 min.
   - Check EHR
   - Stroll - 2 min
   - Brisk walk - 4 min.
3. Cool down stroll 5 min.
4. Stretch (see illustrations)

A.M. SNACK

1 small apple with 1 slice low-fat cheese

Total time - 26 min.
(Do Not Count Cool Down)

LUNCH P/F

spaghetti w/ meat sauce
small tossed salad with
*dressing
or
Tuesday's lunch

2) Mini Tramp

1. Warm up gentle bounce - 4 min.
2. Alternate on and off tramp:
   - Jog in place - 4 min.
   - Walk around room - 2 min.
   - Jog in place - 4 min.
   - Check EHR
   - Walk around room - 2 min.
   - Jog in place - 4 min.
   - Check EHR
   - Walk around room - 2 min.
   - Jog in place - 4 min.
3. Cool down gentle bounce - 5 min.
4. Stretch (see illustrations)

AFTERNOON SNACK

raw veggies w/ 1/3 cup *onion dip

DINNER

*Acidophilus Shake (1/2 before dinner as appetizer)
2-4 oz. skinless chicken or turkey breast
1/2 cup vegetables - green beans or broccoli
(meat, veggies - optional)

Total time - 26 min.
(Do Not Count Cool Down)

EVENING SNACK

raw veggies

How much water today? _____

* See Recipes

How Did You Do?
1) Goal - 26 min.
2) Actual Time _____
3) Goal Reached?   Yes   No
4) EHR? High Low Just Right

Day 5 – Friday

MENU

BREAKFAST
1/2 English muffin w/ 1 tsp. margarine
*hot cereal (amount desired)
4 amino acid tablets

A.M. SNACK
*1/2 cup fat-free yogurt w/ fruit
or
1 small piece fresh raw fruit

LUNCH
sandwich on 2 thin sliced whole grain bread:
1 slice low-fat cheese, lettuce,
1 tbsp. *mayo (optional)
4 hard-boiled egg <u>whites</u>
1 cup soup
carrot and celery strips

AFTERNOON SNACK
3 cups fat-free popcorn w/ Butter Buds powder or 1 tbsp. Parmesan cheese

DINNER
*Acidophilus Shake (1/2 before dinner as appetizer)
3-4 oz. broiled fish
1/2 cup cooked green leafy vegetables, green beans, or broccoli
(meat, veggies - optional)

EVENING SNACK
4 *melba toast with *strawberry jelly
or
raw veggies

How much water today? _____

*   See Recipes

ACTIVITY
1) Walking or 2) Mini Tramp

1) Walking
1. Warm up stroll - 4 min.
2. Alternate brisk walk and stroll:
   - Brisk walk - 4 min.
   - Stroll - 2 min.
   - Brisk walk - 4 min.
   - Check EHR
   - Stroll - 2 min.
   - Brisk walk - 4 min.
   - Check EHR
   - Stroll - 2 min.
   - Brisk walk - 4 min.
3. Cool down stroll 5 min.
4. Stretch (see illustrations)

Total time - 26 min.
(Do Not Count Cool Down)

2) Mini Tramp
1. Warm up gentle bounce - 4 min.
2. Alternate on and off tramp:
   - Jog in place - 4 min.
   - Walk around room - 2 min.
   - Jog in place - 4 min.
   - Check EHR
   - Walk around room - 2 min.
   - Jog in place - 4 min.
   - Check EHR
   - Walk around room - 2 min.
   - Jog in place - 4 min.
3. Cool down gentle bounce - 5 min.
4. Stretch (see illustrations)

Total time - 26 min.
(Do Not Count Cool Down)

How Did You Do?
1) Goal - 26 min.
2) Actual Time _____
3) Goal Reached? Yes No
4) EHR? High Low Just Right

Day 6 – Saturday

MENU	ACTIVITY

ACTIVITY
1) Walking or 2) Mini Tramp

MENU

BREAKFAST
2-4 thin slices *french toast
*fat-free yogurt with fruit -
1/2 cup or more if desired

A.M. SNACK
raw veggies - your choice
or
1 small piece fresh raw fruit

LUNCH
1 cup soup
large tossed salad with
    *dressing
2 whole wheat crackers or
4 *melba toast
4 amino acid tablets

AFTERNOON SNACK
1/2 sandwich - whole grain
bread w/ 1/2 low-fat cheese slice

DINNER
1/2 cup. cooked green veggies
1 small baked potato with 3
tbsp. *"sour cream" or 1 tbsp.
regular sour cream
4-7 oz. baked or broiled fish or
seafood
small tossed salad w/ *dressing

EVENING SNACK
1/8 slice *cheese cake
        or
raw veggies

How much water today?

*   See Recipes

1) Walking
1. Warm up stroll - 4 min.
2. Alternate brisk walk and
    stroll:
    • Brisk walk - 4 min.
    • Stroll - 2 min.
    • Brisk walk - 4 min.
    • Check EHR
    • Stroll - 2 min.
    • Brisk walk - 4 min.
    • Check EHR
    • Stroll - 2 min.
    • Brisk walk - 4 min.
3. Cool down stroll 5 min.
4. Stretch (see illustrations)

    Total time - 26 min.
    (Do Not Count Cool Down)

2) Mini Tramp
1. Warm up gentle bounce - 4
    min.
2. Alternate on and off tramp:
    • Jog in place - 4 min.
    • Walk around room - 2 min.
    • Jog in place - 4 min.
    • Check EHR
    • Walk around room - 2 min.
    • Jog in place - 4 min.
    • Check EHR
    • Walk around room - 2 min.
    • Jog in place - 4 min.
3. Cool down gentle bounce - 5
    min.
4. Stretch (see illustrations)
        Total time - 26 min.
    (Do Not Count Cool Down)

How Did You Do?
1) Goal - 26 min.
2) Actual Time _____
3) Goal Reached?   Yes   No
4) EHR? High Low Just Right

Day 7 – Sunday

MENU	ACTIVITY

ACTIVITY
1) Walking or 2) Mini Tramp

MENU

BREAKFAST
2-4 thin *cinnamon toast
1/2 grapefruit
4 amino acid tablets
or
Have Wednesday's breakfast

A.M. SNACK
*1/2 cup fat-free yogurt w/ fruit
or
raw veggies

LUNCH
1/2 cup cooked veggies
small baked potato or *sweet
potato, or 1/2 cup rice
4-6 oz. baked or broiled lean
meat

AFTERNOON SNACK
1/8 slice *cheese cake
or
raw veggies w/ 1/3 cup *onion
dip

DINNER
1 cup soup
4 *melba toast w/ 1/4 low-fat
cheese slice on each

EVENING SNACK
raw veggies or *Acidophilus
"Snack" Shake

How much water today? _____

*   See Recipes

1) Walking
1. Warm up stroll - 4 min.
2. Alternate brisk walk and
   stroll:
   - Brisk walk - 5 min.
   - Stroll - 2 min.
   - Brisk walk - 5 min.
   - Check EHR
   - Stroll - 2 min.
   - Brisk walk - 5 min.
   - Check EHR
   - Stroll - 2 min.
   - Brisk walk - 5 min.
3. Cool down stroll 5 min.
4. Stretch (see illustrations)

Total time - 30 min.
(Do Not Count Cool Down)

2) Mini Tramp
1. Warm up gentle bounce - 4
   min.
2. Alternate on and off tramp:
   - Jog in place - 5 min.
   - Walk around room - 2 min.
   - Jog in place - 5 min.
   - Check EHR
   - Walk around room - 2 min.
   - Jog in place - 5 min.
   - Check EHR
   - Walk around room - 2 min.
   - Jog in place - 5 min.
3. Cool down gentle bounce - 5
   min.
4. Stretch (see illustrations)
   Total time - 30 min.
   (Do Not Count Cool Down)

How Did You Do?
1) Goal - 30 min.
2) Actual Time _____
3) Goal Reached?   Yes   No
4) EHR? High Low Just Right

Weekly Success Record
Week #2

*Weight

Weight – Day 8 _____   Total lost this week _____
Weight – Day 15 _____   Total lost to date   _____

* Always weigh yourself first thing in the morning without
  clothes or shoes.

Measurements

Day 8	Day 15	Total lost
chest _____	chest _____	_____
waist _____	waist _____	_____
upper rt. thigh _____	upper rt. thigh _____	_____
upper lt. thigh _____	upper lt. thigh _____	_____
hips _____	hips _____	_____

* Inches lost will be more dramatic than pounds lost when you're
  losing body fat. One pound of fat takes up approximately five
  times the space of one pound of lean!

Activity

Goal – 35 minutes by day 14

Day 8 – Total Time _____   Day 14 – Total Time _____

Water

Day 8 – drank _____ cups   Day 9 – drank _____ cups

Day 10 – drank _____ cups   Day 11 – drank _____ cups

Day 12 – drank _____ cups   Day 13 – drank _____ cups

Day 14 – drank _____ cups

Energy Level

(Check One)

Day 8 ___Good ___ Not Good ___ Improving ___ Not Improving

Day 9 ___Good ___ Not Good ___ Improving ___ Not Improving

Day 10 ___Good ___ Not Good ___ Improving ___ Not Improving

Day 11 ___Good ___ Not Good ___ Improving ___ Not Improving

Day 12 ___Good ___ Not Good ___ Improving ___ Not Improving

Day 13 ___Good ___ Not Good ___ Improving ___ Not Improving

Day 14 ___Good ___ Not Good ___ Improving ___ Not Improving

* Anytime you are feeling tired for no apparent reason, and/or you are experiencing real hunger in the evenings, you should *increase* complex carbohydrates. First, increase afternoon snacks – whole grain bagel, popcorn, 1/2-1 sandwich on whole grain bread, etc. If tiredness or evening hunger persists, increase food intake at lunch in addition.

Menus – Weeks Two to Four

Menus for weeks two through four offer two to three choices for each snack and meal, each day. Similar to a restaurant menu, a variety of foods as well as meals are listed that will suit a variety of situations. There are meal choices for eating out, eating at home, or for brown bagging.

This convenience and flexibility, however, should not lead you to deviate from the basic principles of the program. In doing so, you will slow your rate of weight loss. The closer you adhere to the program, including both the Eating Plan *and* Activity Plan, the sooner you will reach your goal.

You may want to use a copier and make a copy of menus to carry with you. This will save you considerable time and trouble, and will also help keep you "on track." Having your own menu to order from avoids a lot of the pitfalls of eating out frequently or unexpectedly.

Breakfasts

Choose one of the breakfasts you want. If you eat breakfast out, either the hot or cold cereal with an English Muffin is available in almost any restaurant. Carry packets of Equal and Butter Buds powder with you. Butter Buds powder may be carried easily in a small empty medicine or vitamin bottle that you've washed and dried well.

A.M. Snacks

Choose one of the morning snacks that you like. A small piece of raw fruit may easily be carried with you for a snack, even if you're traveling. The main thing is to *plan ahead* and take snacks with you. If your breakfast and lunch are only 3 hours apart, you may skip this snack if you wish, after week I.

Lunches

The microwave plate that you fix the night before (see #21 "Weight Loss Special Notes") will be excellent if you have access to a microwave at lunchtime. If not, there are choices on the menus for either packing a lunch or eating in a restaurant. Have one of the lunches that suits you best.

Afternoon Snacks

This snack is the most important of all. *Never* omit the afternoon snack! If you have as much as six hours between lunch and dinner, it may be wise to add a second afternoon snack: 1) one raw vegetable snack *early* afternoon, and 2) your regular snack *late* afternoon. Choose a snack that you like and is convenient for your particular situation.

Dinner

If you live alone, or if your family is not at home for dinner, the Acidophilus Shake is convenient and easy to prepare. With approximately 30 grams of high quality protein and practically no fat, it is also a very healthy drink.

If you and your family usually eat dinner together you should continue to eat with them. Simply have 1/2 of the Shake as an appetizer and the other 1/2 with child-sized portions of whatever food has been prepared for the family, with the exception of dessert. If they're having dessert, save half of your shake for your dessert. (See "Weight Loss Special Notes," #21.)

If you eat dinner out, there are meals listed to choose from every night of the week. It is important that you get into the habit of asking for a "doggie bag." You've paid for the food – why waste it? Take leftover food in a doggie bag and have it for lunch the next day. Some of my best lunches have come from those convenient "doggie bags"! And what a compliment to the restaurant – their food is so good that you can't resist taking it with you! Or if you wish, visit one of the many restaurants offering soup and salad bars. Take advantage of this excellent evening meal. Just remember to have only the veggies, and prepare your own dressing as described in the Recipe section – very tasty and simple to do when eating out.

Remember, poultry, seafood and fish (#20 "Weight Loss Special Notes") are the best selections, especially for dinner meats! This does not mean you cannot have others *occasionally*.

P.M. Snacks

Choose one evening snack to be eaten any time after dinner that you wish. The nice thing about these snacks is they help keep you from overeating at dinner because you know there's always an evening snack waiting for you after dinner. If something sweet tasting is what you occasionally must have in the evening, check the list of more than twenty items in the "Good For You Sweets" section of the "Special Helps" chapter.

Week 2

I. Beginning Weight and Measurements

Weigh yourself in the morning, nude, and record weight on both your Master Success Record, and Weekly Success Record. After recording weight, measure with a snug, not tight, measuring tape and record as indicated on Master Success Record and Weekly Success Record.

II. Activity Plan

Read over Activity Plan for day #8. If you are not ready to increase as indicated, remain at Week I level. If you need to increase *more*, go to Week 3 level. Be sure to read chapter on stretching.

III. Eating Plan

A. Read over this week's menu and list groceries you need.
B. List recipes you will be using for the week and make sure you include ingredients needed on your grocery list.
C. Make any recipes that you can ahead of time.
D. The word "meat" on menus also includes poultry, fish, and seafood.
E. Re-read "Weight Loss Special Notes."

Day 8 - Monday

BREAKFASTS
1. 1 WW toast w/ 1 slice low-fat cheese, melted (#22 "Weight Loss Special Notes" - low-fat cheese)
2. 1/2 English Muffin w/ 1 tsp. margarine
   *hot cereal
   4 amino acid tablets

A.M. SNACKS
1. 1 small piece raw fruit
2. raw veggies

LUNCHES
1. microwave plate from last night's dinner (#21 "Weight Loss Special Notes")
2. 5-6 oz. lean meat
   small baked potato w/ 1 tsp. margarine or 1 tbsp. sour cream
   tossed salad and/or cooked veggie
3. 5-6 oz. lean meat on 2 thin sliced whole grain bread w/ lettuce, tomato (1 tbsp. *mayo, optional)
   1 cup soup (optional)
   1/2 large salt-free pretzel

*   See Recipes

AFTERNOON SNACKS
1. 1 slice whole grain bread
   2 tsp. peanut butter
2. 1 small baked potato w/ 1/4 cup *"sour cream"
3. 1 whole grain bagel

DINNERS
1. *Acidophilus Shake
2. *Acidophilus Shake (have 1/2 as appetizer before dinner)
   Child-sized portions of family's dinner (see #21 "Weight Loss Special Notes")
3.** large tossed salad w/ *dressing
   1 cup soup (optional)
   4 amino acid tablets
4.** tossed salads* (2 small):
   1st before meal as appetizer
   2nd eat with meal (*dressing)
   4 oz. fish or seafood
   small serving non seed-type veggies

**   (Use #3 or #4 if eating dinner out. "Doggie-bag" extra food, if any, for lunch tomorrow.)

P.M. SNACKS
1. raw veggies or *sweet cucumbers
2. 1/2 cup fat-free *yogurt w/ fruit

ACTIVITY - WALKING OR MINI TRAMP

WALKING
1. Warm up stroll 4 min.
2. Alternate: 8 min. brisk walk, 2 min. stroll to total 25 min. Check EHR.
3. Cool down stroll 5 min.
4. Stretch
5. Total time without warm up 30 min.

MINI TRAMP
1. Warm up gentle bounce 4 min.
2. Alternate: 8 min. on tramp, 2 min. off tramp to total 25 min. Check EHR.
3. Cool down stroll 5 min.
4. Stretch
5. Total time without warm up 30 min.

Goal - 30 min.
Actual Time _____   Goal Reached? _____   EHR? High Low OK

Day 9 - Tuesday

BREAKFASTS
1. *Egg and cheese muffin
2. *Hot cereal
   1 whole grain toast
   1 tsp. margarine
   4 amino acid tablets
3. 1 whole grain toast w/* jelly
   1/2 cup sugar-free cold cereal
   1/2 cup fat-free milk
   4 amino acid tablets

A.M. SNACKS
1. 1 small piece raw fruit
2. *1/2 cup fat-free yogurt w/ fruit

LUNCHES
1. microwave plate from last
   night's dinner
2. 5-6 oz. poultry or fish
   1 whole grain bread or roll
   cooked veggies
3. 2/3-1 cup *tuna salad on
   lettuce w/ 1/2 tomato
   1 large salt-free pretzel
   1 cup soup (optional)

*   See Recipes

AFTERNOON SNACKS
1. 1 small baked potato w/ 1/4
   cup *"sour cream"
2. popcorn - fat-free, 3 cups
   sprinkled with Butter Buds
   powder
3. 1/2 sandwich - 1 whole grain
   bread w/ 1/2 slice low-fat cheese

DINNERS
1. *Acidophilus Shake
2. *Acidophilus Shake (1/2 as
   appetizer before dinner)
   Child-sized portion of
   family's dinner
3. 1-2 cups soup ("Weight Loss
   Special Notes" #17)
   2 wasa w/ 1 thin slice
   Farmer's Cheese on each
4. **tossed salads* (2 small):
   1st before meal as appetizer
   2nd eat w/ meal (*dressing)
   4 oz. fish or seafood
   small serving non seed-type
   veggies

**   (Use #4 if eating dinner out.
   "Doggie bag" extra food, if
   any, for lunch tomorrow.)

P.M. SNACKS
1. raw veggies or 1 cup *slaw
2. *Acidophilus "Snack" Shake

ACTIVITY - WALKING OR MINI TRAMP

WALKING
1. Warm up stroll 4 min.
2. Alternate: <u>8 min</u>. brisk walk,
   <u>2 min</u>. stroll to total 25 min.
   Check EHR.
3. Cool down stroll 5 min.
4. Stretch (see illustrations)
5. Total time without warm up
   30 min.

MINI TRAMP
1. Warm up gentle bounce 4 min.
2. Alternate: <u>8 min</u>. on tramp,
   <u>2 min</u>. off tramp to total 25
   min. Check EHR.
3. Cool down stroll 5 min.
4. Stretch (see illustrations)
5. Total time without warm up
   30 min.

Goal - 30 min.
Actual Time _____   Goal Reached? _____   EHR? High Low OK

Day 10 - Wednesday

BREAKFASTS
1. 1 whole grain toast w/ *jelly
   1/2 cup sugar-free cold cereal
   1/2 cup fat-free milk
   4 amino acid tablets
2. 1/2 English Muffin w/ 1 tsp. margarine
   *hot cereal
   4 amino acid tablets
3. 2-4 thin whole grain *cinnamon toast
   1/2 cup low-fat cottage cheese w/ unsweetened peaches

A.M. SNACKS
1. 1 small piece raw fruit
2. celery w/ 2 tbsp. Light Cream Cheese

LUNCHES
1. microwave plate from last night's dinner
2. 5-6 oz. lean meat
   1/3 cup rice or 1 small baked potato w/ 1 tsp. margarine cooked veggies
3. 4-5 oz. skinless chicken breast on 2 thin-sliced whole grain bread w/ lettuce, tomato (1 tbsp. *mayo, optional)
   1 cup soup (optional)
   1 wasa or 1/2 large salt-free pretzel

* See Recipes

AFTERNOON SNACKS
1. 1 whole grain bagel
2. raw veggies w/ 1/3 cup *onion dip
3. 1/2 sandwich - 1 whole grain bread w/ 1/4 cup *egg salad

DINNERS
1. *Acidophilus Shake
   (1/2 for appetizer before dinner)
   Child-sized portions of family's dinner (optional)
2. Chef's Salad w *dressing - use 1 1/2 slices low-fat cheese plus 3 hard boiled egg whites only
   2 oz. chicken breast
   1 wasa, rice cake, or 4 *melba
3.** large tossed salad w/ *dressing
   1 cup soup (optional)
   4 amino acid tablets
4.** 1 cup soup (not creamed) before meal - appetizer
   4 oz. fish or seafood
   small serving non seed-type veggies
   small tossed salad (optional)

** (Use #3 or #4 if eating dinner out. "Doggie bag" extra food, if any, for lunch tomorrow.)

P.M. SNACKS
1. raw veggies or *sweet cucumbers
2. 2 *fudgesicles

ACTIVITY - WALKING OR MINI TRAMP

WALKING
1. Warm up stroll 4 min.
2. Alternate: 8 min. brisk walk, 2 min. stroll to total 30 min. Check EHR.
3. Cool down stroll 5 min.
4. Stretch (see illustrations)
5. Total time without warm up 35 min.

MINI TRAMP
1. Warm up gentle bounce 4 min.
2. Alternate: 8 min. on tramp, 2 min. off tramp to total 30 min. Check EHR.
3. Cool down stroll 5 min.
4. Stretch (see illustrations)
5. Total time without warm up 35 min.

Goal - 35 min.
Actual Time ———— Goal Reached? ———— EHR? High Low OK

Day 11 - Thursday

BREAKFASTS

1. *Bagel Breakfast "Danish
2. 1/2 English Muffin w/ 1 tsp. margarine
   *hot cereal
   4 amino acid tablets
3. 1/2 bagel, toasted w/ 2 tbsp.
   *Whipped Light Cream Cheese
   1/2 cup sugar-free cold cereal
   1/2 cup fat-free milk

A.M. SNACKS

1. 1 cup light soup
2. *1/2 cup fat-free yogurt w/ fruit

LUNCHES

1. microwave plate from last night's dinner
2. 2/3-1 cup *Tuna or *Chicken salad on lettuce w/ 1/2 tomato
   1 large salt-free pretzel
3. 5-6 oz. lean meat
   1/3 cup rice or small baked potato
   cooked veggies

* See Recipes

AFTERNOON SNACK

1. popcorn, fat-free, 3 cups sprinkled w/ Butter Buds powder
2. 1 small baked potato
3. 1/2 sandwich - 1 whole grain bread, 2 tsp. peanut butter (*jelly optional)

DINNERS

1. *Acidophilus Shake
2. *Acidophilus Shake (1/2 before dinner as appetizer)
   child-sized portions of family's dinner foods
3.** large tossed salad w/ *dressing
   1 cup soup (optional)
   4 amino acid tablets
4.** tossed salads (2 small):
   1st before meal - appetizer
   2nd eat w/ meal (*dressing)
   4 oz. skinless chicken or turkey breast
   small serving non seed-type veggies

** (Use #3 or #4 if eating dinner out. "Doggie bag" extra food, if any, for lunch tomorrow.)

P.M. SNACKS

1. raw veggies
2. *jello w/ 1/4 cup cottage cheese

ACTIVITY - WALKING OR MINI TRAMP

WALKING

1. Warm up stroll 4 min.
2. Alternate: 8 min. brisk walk, 2 min. stroll to total 30 min. Check EHR.
3. Cool down stroll 5 min.
4. Stretch
5. Total time without warm up 35 min.

MINI TRAMP

1. Warm up gentle bounce 4 min.
2. Alternate: 8 min. on tramp, 2 min. off tramp to total 30 min. Check EHR.
3. Cool down stroll 5 min.
4. Stretch
5. Total time without warm up 35 min.

Goal - 35 min.
Actual Time _____   Goal Reached? _____   EHR? High Low OK

Day 12 - Friday

BREAKFASTS
1. Thin sliced Farmer's Cheese, melted on 1/2 English Muffin 1/2 cup sugar-free cold cereal w/ 1/2 cup fat-free milk
2. 1/2 bagel w/ 1 tsp. margarine *hot cereal 4 amino acid tablets
3. 2-4 thin whole grain *cinnamon toast 1/2 cup *yogurt w/ Grape Nuts

A.M. SNACKS
1. 1 small piece raw fruit
2. celery w/ 3 tbsp. *Whipped Light Cream Cheese

LUNCHES
1. microwave plate from last night's dinner
2. 5-6 oz. lean meat 1 small baked potato or 1 bread w/ 1 tsp. margarine veggies - cooked or raw
3. *egg salad w/ lettuce on 2 thin-sliced whole grain bread 1 cup soup

* See Recipes

AFTERNOON SNACKS
1. 1 whole grain bagel
2. 1/2 sandwich - 1 whole grain bread w/ 1/2 slice low-fat cheese
3. *Waldorf Salad

DINNERS
1. *Acidophilus Shake
2. *Acidophilus Shake (1/2 before dinner as appetizer) child-sized portions of family's dinner foods
3.** 4-6 oz. fish or seafood 1/2 small baked potato or 1 thin sliced bread small serving non seed-type veggies
4.** large tossed salad w/ *dressing 1 cup soup (optional) 4 amino acid tablets

** (Use #3 or #4 if eating dinner out. "Doggie bag" extra food, if any, for lunch tomorrow.)

P.M. SNACKS
1. raw veggies w/ 1/4 cup *Ranch dressing or *onion dip
2. *cucumbers - sweet
3. 1/8 slice *cheese cake

ACTIVITY - WALKING OR MINI TRAMP

WALKING
1. Warm up stroll 4 min.
2. Alternate: 8 min. brisk walk, 2 min. stroll to total 30 min. Check EHR.
3. Cool down stroll 5 min.
4. Stretch (see illustrations)
5. Total time without warm up 35 min.

MINI TRAMP
1. Warm up gentle bounce 4 min.
2. Alternate: 8 min. on tramp, 2 min. off tramp to total 30 min. Check EHR.
3. Cool down stroll 5 min.
4. Stretch (see illustrations)
5. Total time without warm up 35 min.

Goal - 35 min.
Actual Time _____   Goal Reached? _____   EHR? High Low OK

Day 13 - Saturday

BREAKFASTS
1. 4-5 pancakes w/ *syrup or *jelly
   1/2 grapefruit
2. *scrambled eggs or *omelet
   2 slices WW toast (1 tsp. margarine on each)
   2 slices Canadian bacon
3. *Bagel breakfast "Danish"
   1/2 grapefruit

A.M. SNACKS
1. 1 small piece raw fruit
2. raw veggies

LUNCHES
1. large tossed salad w/ *dressing
   1 cup soup
   4 amino acid tablets
2. Chef's salad:
   2 egg whites
   1 1/2 slices low-fat cheese
   3 oz. skinless chicken breast
   *dressing (optional)
3. 4 oz. (lean only) roast beef in sandwich w/ lettuce, 1 tbsp.
   *mayo or mustard on 2 thin-sliced whole grain bread
   1 cup soup or small tossed salad w/ *dressing

*   See Recipes

AFTERNOON SNACKS
1. 1/2 bagel w/ 2 tbsp.
   *Whipped Light Cream Cheese
2. 1/2 sandwich - 1 hard boiled egg white, 1/2 slice low-fat cheese
3. raw veggies w/ 1/3 cup *onion dip

DINNERS
1. *Acidophilus Shake
2. *Acidophilus Shake (1/2 before dinner as appetizer)
   2 oz. skinless chicken breast, fish or seafood
   2/3 cup cooked non seed-type veggies
3.** 4 oz. skinless chicken breast, fish or seafood
   1/2 small baked potato
   cooked non seed-type veggies or tossed salad w/ *dressing (small)
4.** large tossed salad w/ *dressing
   1 cup soup (optional)
   4 amino acid tablets

** (Use #3 or #4 if eating dinner out. "Doggie bag" extra food, if any, for lunch tomorrow.)

P.M. SNACKS
1. 1/8 slice *cheese cake
2. raw veggies
3. 1 1/2 cup popcorn - fat free w/ Butter Buds

ACTIVITY - WALKING OR MINI TRAMP

WALKING
1. Warm up stroll 4 min.
2. Alternate: <u>8 min.</u> brisk walk, <u>2 min.</u> stroll to total 30 min. Check EHR.
3. Cool down stroll 5 min.
4. Stretch (see illustrations)
5. Total time without warm up 35 min.

Goal - 35 min.

MINI TRAMP
1. Warm up gentle bounce 4 min.
2. Alternate: <u>8 min.</u> on tramp, <u>2 min.</u> off tramp to total 30 min. Check EHR.
3. Cool down stroll 5 min.
4. Stretch (see illustrations)
5. Total time without warm up 35 min.

Actual Time _____   Goal Reached? _____   EHR? High Low OK

Day 14 - Sunday

BREAKFASTS
1. 4-5 pancakes w/ *syrup or *jelly
   3 slices Canadian bacon
   1/2 grapefruit
2. *scrambled eggs or *omelet
   2 WW toast (1 tsp. margarine on
   each)
   2 slices Canadian bacon
3. raisin bagel - split w/ 2 tbsp.
   *Whipped Light Cream
   Cheese on each half, topped
   w/ *jelly

A.M. SNACKS
1. 1 fresh or 1 cup sugar-free
   peaches
2. raw veggies

LUNCHES
1. 3 oz. lean baked ham
   small *sweet potato
   1 vegetable
   small tossed salad, *dressing
2. 5-6 oz. lean broiled steak
   1 small baked potato w/ 1
   tbsp. sour cream
   small *tossed salad
   (*dressing) or cooked veggie
3. *Tuna Melt
   small tossed salad w/ *dressing

*   See Recipes

AFTERNOON SNACKS
1. 3 cups popcorn - fat-free w/
   Butter Buds powder
2. 1/2 sandwich w/ 1/2 slice
   low-fat cheese
3. raw veggies w/ 1/3 cup
   *onion dip

DINNERS
1. *Acidophilus Shake
2.** large tossed salad w/ *dressing
   1 cup soup (optional)
   4 amino acid tablets
3. 1 thin-sliced whole grain
   toast w/ 2 thin slices
   Farmer's Cheese, melted
   1 cup soup
   small tossed salad w/ *dressing
4.** 1 bowl vegetable soup
   2 whole grain crackers
   4 amino acid tablets

**   (Use #2 or #4 if eating dinner
       out. "Doggie bag" extra food,
       if any, for lunch tomorrow.)

P.M. SNACKS
1. 2 *fudgesicles
2. raw veggies
3. 1/2 cup fat-free *yogurt w/
   Grape Nuts or Nuggets

ACTIVITY - WALKING OR MINI TRAMP

WALKING
1. Warm up stroll 4 min.
2. Alternate: <u>8 min</u>. brisk walk,
   <u>2 min</u>. stroll to total 30 min.
   Check EHR.
3. Cool down stroll 5 min.
4. Stretch (see illustrations)
5. Total time without warm up
   35 min.

MINI TRAMP
1. Warm up gentle bounce 4 min.
2. Alternate: <u>8 min</u>. on tramp,
   <u>2 min.</u> off tramp to total 30
   min. Check EHR.
3. Cool down stroll 5 min.
4. Stretch (see illustrations)
5. Total time without warm up
   35 min.

Goal - 35 min.
Actual Time ———   Goal Reached?———   EHR? High Low OK

Weekly Success Record
Week #3

*Weight

Weight – Day 15 _____   Total lost this week _____
Weight – Day 22 _____   Total lost to date   _____

* Always weigh yourself first thing in the morning without clothes or shoes.

Measurements

Day 15	Day 22	Total lost
chest _____	chest _____	_____
waist _____	waist _____	_____
upper rt. thigh _____	upper rt. thigh _____	_____
upper lt. thigh _____	upper lt. thigh _____	_____
hips _____	hips _____	_____

* Inches lost will be more dramatic than pounds lost when you're losing body fat. One pound of fat takes up approximately five times the space of one pound of lean!

Activity

Goal – 40 minutes by day 21

Day 15 – Total Time _____   Day 21 – Total Time _____

Water

Day 15 – drank _____ cups   Day 16 – drank _____ cups

Day 17 – drank _____ cups   Day 18 – drank _____ cups

Day 19 – drank _____ cups   Day 20 – drank _____ cups

Day 21 – drank _____ cups

Energy Level

(Check One)

Day 15 ____ Good ____ Not Good ____ Improving ____ Not Improving

Day 16 ____ Good ____ Not Good ____ Improving ____ Not Improving

Day 17 ____ Good ____ Not Good ____ Improving ____ Not Improving

Day 18 ____ Good ____ Not Good ____ Improving ____ Not Improving

Day 19 ____ Good ____ Not Good ____ Improving ____ Not Improving

Day 20 ____ Good ____ Not Good ____ Improving ____ Not Improving

Day 21 ____ Good ____ Not Good ____ Improving ____ Not Improving

* Anytime you are feeling tired for no apparent reason, and/or you are experiencing real hunger in the evenings, you should *increase* complex carbohydrates. First, increase afternoon snacks – whole grain bagel, popcorn, 1/2-1 sandwich on whole grain bread, etc. If tiredness or evening hunger persists, increase food intake at lunch in addition.

Week 3

I. Beginning Weight and Measurements

Weigh yourself in the morning, nude, and record weight on both your Master Success Record, and Weekly Success Record. After recording weight, measure with a snug, not tight, measuring tape and record as indicated on Master Success Record, and Weekly Success Record.

II. Activity Plan

Read over Activity Plan for day 15. If you are not ready to increase as indicated, remain at week 2 level. If you need to increase *more*, go to week 4 level. Be sure to read chapter on stretching.

III. Eating Plan

A. Read over this week's menu and list groceries you need.
B. List recipes you will be using for the week and make sure you include ingredients needed on your grocery list.
C. Make any recipes that you can ahead of time.
D. The word "meat" on menu also includes poultry, fish and seafood
E. Re-read "Weight Loss Special Notes."

Day 15 - Monday

BREAKFASTS
1. 1/2 English Muffin w/ 1 slice low-fat cheese, melted 1/2 cup sugar-free cold cereal w/ 1/2 cup fat-free milk
2. *Breakfast-In-A-Muffin
3. *hot cereal 1 whole grain toast w/ *jelly 4 amino acid tablets

A.M. SNACKS
1. 1 small piece raw fruit
2. 1/2 cup fat-free *yogurt w/ fruit

LUNCHES
1. *chili raw veggies or tossed salad w/ *dressing
2. 2/3-1 cup *tuna salad on lettuce w/ 1/2 tomato 1/2 large salt-free pretzel 1 cup soup (optional)
3. 5-6 oz. lean meat cooked veggies 1 whole grain bread or roll

*   See Recipes

AFTERNOON SNACKS
1. 1/2 whole grain bagel w/ 2 tsp. peanut butter
2. 1 small baked potato w/ slice low-fat cheese
3. 1/2 sandwich - 1 whole grain bread w/ low-fat cheese

DINNERS
1. Chef's salad: 3 oz. white tuna 1 hard boiled egg white 1 slice low-fat cheese 1/3 cup low-fat cottage cheese any raw veggies desired
2. *Acidophilus Shake (1/2 before dinner as appetizer) child-sized portions of family's dinner foods
3.** large tossed salad w/ *dressing 1 cup soup (optional)
4.** 4 oz. skinless chicken or turkey 1/2 baked or boiled potato(small) 1/3 cup cooked non seed-type veggies

** (Use #3 or #4 if eating dinner out. "Doggie bag" extra food, if any, for lunch tomorrow.)

P.M. SNACKS
1. raw veggies or 1 cup *slaw
2. 1/2 cup low-fat cottage cheese w/ fresh or unsweetened peach half

---

ACTIVITY - WALKING OR MINI TRAMP

WALKING
1. Warm up stroll 4 min.
2. Alternate: 10 min. brisk walk, 2 min. stroll to total 35 min. Check EHR.
3. Cool down stroll 5 min.
4. Stretch (see illustrations)
5. Total time without warm up 40 min.

Goal - 40 min.

MINI TRAMP
1. Warm up gentle bounce 4 min.
2. Alternate: 10 min. on tramp, 2 min. off tramp to total 35 min. Check EHR.
3. Cool down stroll 5 min.
4. Stretch (see illustrations)
5. Total time without warm up 40 min.

Actual Time ———   Goal Reached? ———   EHR? High Low OK

Day 16 - Tuesday

BREAKFASTS
1. 1/2 bagel w/ thin slices
   Farmer's Cheese, melted
   *yogurt w/ fruit
2. *hot cereal
   1 whole grain toast
   4 amino acid tablets
3. *Breakfast Bagel "Danish"

A.M. SNACKS
1. 1 small piece raw fruit
2. raw veggies

LUNCHES
1. regular pizza 1-2 slices or
   1 whole "Tony's Microlite
   Pizza" (a low-fat pan-size pizza)
   small tossed salad w/ *dressing
2. 4-5 oz. lean roast beef on 2
   thin WW bread w/ lettuce,
   mustard or 1 tbsp. *mayo, or
   horseradish
   1 cup soup
3. microwave plate from last
   night's dinner

*   See Recipes

AFTERNOON SNACKS
1. 1/2 sandwich - 1 whole grain
   bread w/ 1/4 cup *egg salad
2. small baked potato w/ 1 low-
   fat cheese slice
3. 1/2 bagel w/ 2 tbsp.
   *Whipped Light Cream
   Cheese or 1 whole bagel, plain

DINNERS
1. *Acidophilus Shake
2. *Acidophilus Shake (1/2
   before dinner as appetizer)
   child-sized portions of
   family's dinner foods
3.** small tossed salads (2)
   1st - before dinner as
   appetizer
   2nd with meal (*dressing)
   1 small skinless chicken
   breast or 2 skinless drumsticks
   small serving non seed-type
   veggies
4.** large tossed salad w/ *dressing
   1 cup soup (optional)
   4 amino acid tablets

**   (Use #3 or #4 if eating dinner
   out. "Doggie bag" extra food,
   if any, for lunch tomorrow.)

P.M. SNACKS
1. raw veggies w/ 1/4 cup
   *onion dip
2. 1/2 small can white tuna
   (canned in water) w/ 3
   *melba toast

ACTIVITY - WALKING OR MINI TRAMP

WALKING
1. Warm up stroll 4 min.
2. Alternate: <u>10 min.</u> brisk walk,
   <u>2 min.</u> stroll to total 35 min.
   Check EHR.
3. Cool down stroll 5 min.
4. Stretch (see illustrations)
5. Total time without warm up
   40 min.

MINI TRAMP
1. Warm up gentle bounce 4 min.
2. Alternate: <u>10 min.</u> on tramp,
   <u>2 min.</u> off tramp to total 35
   min. Check EHR.
3. Cool down stroll 5 min.
4. Stretch (see illustrations)
5. Total time without warm up
   40 min.

Goal - 40 min.
Actual Time _____   Goal Reached?_____   EHR? High Low OK

Day 17 - Wednesday

BREAKFASTS
1. 1/2 cup sugar-free cold cereal
   1/2 cup fat-free milk
   1 whole grain toast w/ 2 thin
   slices Farmer's Cheese, melted
2. *hot cereal
   1 WW toast w/ 1 tsp
   margarine and *jelly (optional)
   4 amino acid tablets
3. 4 *pancakes w/ *syrup or *jelly
   1/2 grapefruit
   4 amino acid tablets

A.M. SNACKS
1. 1 cup lite soup
2. raw veggies

LUNCHES
1. microwave plate from last
   night's dinner
2. 5-6 oz. lean meat
   1/3 cup steamed veggies
   small baked potato (optional)
3. 5 oz. lean meat in sandwich
   w/ 2 thin slices WW bread,
   lettuce, tomato, 1 tbsp.
   *mayo (optional)
   1 cup soup

*   See Recipes

AFTERNOON SNACKS
1. 3 cups popcorn w/ Butter
   Buds powder or 1 tbsp.
   Parmesan cheese
2. 1/2 sandwich w/ 2 tsp.
   peanut butter, *jelly
3. 1/2 cup *rice pudding

DINNERS
1. *Acidophilus Shake
2. *Acidophilus Shake (1/2
   before dinner as appetizer)
   child-sized portions of
   family's dinner foods
3.** 4 oz. fish
   1/2 small potato
   small tossed salad w/ *dressing
4.** large tossed salad w/
   *dressing
   1 cup soup (optional)
   4 amino acid tablets

**   (Use #3 or #4 if eating dinner
   out. "Doggie bag" extra food,
   if any, for lunch tomorrow.)

P.M. SNACKS
1. raw veggies
2. 4 *melba toast w/ *jelly
3. 2 *melba toast w/ 1 tsp.
   peanut butter

ACTIVITY - WALKING OR MINI TRAMP

WALKING
1. Warm up stroll 4 min.
2. Alternate: <u>10 min</u>. brisk walk,
   <u>2 min</u>. stroll to total 35 min.
   Check EHR.
3. Cool down stroll 5 min.
4. Stretch (see illustrations)
5. Total time without warm up
   40 min.

MINI TRAMP
1. Warm up gentle bounce
   4 min.
2. Alternate: <u>10 min</u>. on
   tramp,
   <u>2 min.</u> off tramp to total
   35 min. Check EHR.
3. Cool down stroll 5 min.
4. Stretch (see illustrations)
5. Total time without warm up
   40 min.

Goal - 40 min.
Actual Time _____   Goal Reached?_____   EHR? High Low OK

Day 18 - Thursday

BREAKFASTS
1. 2-4 thin whole grain
   *cinnamon toast
   1/2 cup *yogurt w/ fruit
2. 1 whole grain toast w/ 1 slice
   low-fat cheese, melted
   *hot cereal
   4 amino acid tablets
3. *omelet
   2 whole grain toast w/ 1 tsp.
   margarine on each
   2 slices Canadian bacon

A.M. SNACKS
1. 1 small piece raw fruit
2. celery w/ 3 tbsp. *Whipped
   Light Cream Cheese

LUNCHES
1. microwave plate from last
   night's dinner
2. 2 cups *Beef or *Chicken Stew
   1 thin sliced whole grain bread
3. 5 oz. lean meat on 2 thin
   sliced whole grain bread w/
   lettuce, (1 tbsp. *mayo optional)
   1 cup soup

*   See Recipes

AFTERNOON SNACKS
1. 3 cups popcorn w/ Butter
   Buds powder or 1 tbsp.
   Parmesan cheese
2. 1/2 sandwich w/ 1/4 cup
   *Egg Salad
3. 1 whole grain bagel

DINNERS
1. *Acidophilus Shake
2. *Acidophilus Shake (1/2
   before dinner as appetizer)
   child-sized portions of
   family's dinner foods
3.** 2 skinless chicken drumsticks
   or 1 small skinless chicken
   breast
   1/4 cup rice
   small tossed salad w/ *dressing
4.** large tossed salad w/ *dressing
   1 cup soup (optional)
   4 amino acid tablets

**   (Use #3 or #4 if eating dinner
   out. "Doggie bag" extra food,
   if any, for lunch tomorrow.)

P.M. SNACKS
1. raw veggies w/ 1/4 cup
   *onion dip
2. 1/3 cup low-fat cottage
   cheese w/ sugar-free
   strawberries
3. 2 pieces *fudge

ACTIVITY - WALKING OR MINI TRAMP

WALKING
1. Warm up stroll 4 min.
2. Alternate: <u>10 min</u>. brisk walk,
   <u>2 min</u>. stroll to total 35 min.
   Check EHR.
3. Cool down stroll 5 min.
4. Stretch (see illustrations)
5. Total time without warm up
   40 min.

MINI TRAMP
1. Warm up gentle bounce 4 min.
2. Alternate: <u>10 min</u>. on tramp,
   <u>2 min</u>. off tramp to total 35
   min. Check EHR.
3. Cool down stroll 5 min.
4. Stretch (see illustrations)
5. Total time without warm up
   40 min.

Goal - 40 min.
Actual Time _____   Goal Reached? _____   EHR? High Low OK

Day 19 - Friday

BREAKFASTS
1. 1 whole grain toast w/ *jelly
   *hot cereal
   4 amino acid tablets
2. 1/2 cup sugar-free cold cereal
   1/2 cup fat-free milk
   1 whole grain toast w/ 2 thin
   slices Farmer's Cheese, melted
3. 1 English Muffin w/ 1/2 slice
   low-fat cheese melted on
   each half
   2/3 cup *yogurt w/ fruit

A.M. SNACKS
1. 1 small piece raw fruit
2. 2 pieces *melba toast w/ 1/4
   slice low-fat cheese on each

LUNCHES
1. microwave plate from last
   night's dinner
2. *egg salad w/ lettuce on 2
   thin sliced whole grain bread
   1 cup soup
3. 5-6 oz. lean meat
   1 small potato or 1 bread w/
   1 tsp margarine
   veggies - cooked or raw -
   small serving

* See Recipes

AFTERNOON SNACKS
1. 1/2 cup *rice pudding
2. 1/2 sandwich - 1 whole grain
   bread w/ 1/2 slice low-fat cheese
3. *Waldorf Salad

DINNERS
1. *Acidophilus Shake
2. *Acidophilus Shake (1/2
   before dinner as appetizer)
   child-sized portions of
   family's dinner foods
3.** 4-6 oz. fish or seafood
   1/2 small potato or 1/4 cup rice
   small serving non seed-type
   veggies, or small tossed
   salad w/ *dressing
4.** large tossed salad w/*dressing
   1 cup soup (optional)
   4 amino acid tablets

** (Use #3 or #4 if eating dinner
   out. "Doggie bag" extra food,
   if any, for lunch tomorrow.)

P.M. SNACKS
1. raw veggies w/ 1/4 cup
   *ranch dressing or *onion dip
2. 3 fudgesicles
3. 1/2 can white tuna (canned
   in water) w/ 3 *melba toast

ACTIVITY - WALKING OR MINI TRAMP

WALKING
1. Warm up stroll 4 min.
2. Alternate: 10 min. brisk walk,
   2 min. stroll to total 35 min.
   Check EHR.
3. Cool down stroll 5 min.
4. Stretch (see illustrations)
5. Total time without warm up
   40 min.

MINI TRAMP
1. Warm up gentle bounce 4 min.
2. Alternate: 10 min. on tramp,
   2 min. off tramp to total 35
   min. Check EHR.
3. Cool down stroll 5 min.
4. Stretch (see illustrations)
5. Total time without warm up
   40 min.

Goal - 40 min.
Actual Time _____   Goal Reached? _____   EHR? High Low OK

Day 20 - Saturday

BREAKFASTS
1. 4-5 *pancakes w/ *syrup or *jelly
   3 slices Canadian bacon
   1/2 grapefruit
2. *Breakfast-In-A-Muffin
3. 1 thin sliced whole grain toast w/ *jelly and 1 tsp. margarine
   *hot cereal
   4 amino acid tablets

A.M. SNACKS
1. 1 small piece raw fruit
2. 1/2 cup *yogurt w/ fruit

LUNCHES
1. large tossed salad w/ *dressing
   1 cup soup (optional)
   4 amino acid tablets
2. large bowl soup (not creamed)
   2 WW crackers
   4 amino acid tablets
3. 4 oz. (lean only) roast beef in sandwich w/ lettuce, 1 tbsp. *mayo, mustard or horseradish on 2 thin slices whole grain bread
   1 cup soup

* See Recipes

AFTERNOON SNACKS
1. 1 bagel
2. 1/2 sandwich - 1 hard boiled egg white, 1/2 slice low-fat cheese
3. 3 cups fat-free popcorn w/ Butter Buds powder

DINNERS
1. *Acidophilus Shake
2. *Acidophilus Shake (1/2 before dinner as appetizer)
   child-sized portions of family's dinner foods
3.** 4-6 oz. skinless chicken, turkey, fish or seafood
   1/2 small baked potato or 1/4 cup rice
   cooked non seed-type veggies or
   tossed salad w/ *dressing
4.** large tossed salad w/ *dressing
   1 cup soup (optional)
   4 amino acid tablets

** (Use #3 or #4 if eating dinner out. "Doggie bag" extra food, if any, for lunch tomorrow.)

P.M. SNACKS
1. 2 fudgesicles
2. 1 piece *Carrot Cake Squares (w/ 1 tbsp. *Whipped Light Cream Cheese - optional)
3. 11/2 cup fat-free popcorn w/ Butter Buds powder

ACTIVITY - WALKING OR MINI TRAMP

WALKING
1. Warm up stroll 4 min.
2. Alternate: <u>10 min</u>. brisk walk, <u>2 min</u>. stroll to total 35 min. Check EHR.
3. Cool down stroll 5 min.
4. Stretch
5. Total time without warm up 40 min.

MINI TRAMP
1. Warm up gentle bounce 4 min.
2. Alternate: <u>10 min</u>. on tramp, <u>2 min</u>. off tramp to total 35 min. Check EHR.
3. Cool down stroll 5 min.
4. Stretch
5. Total time without warm up 40 min.

Goal - 40 min.
Actual Time_____   Goal Reached?_____   EHR? High Low OK

Day 21 - Sunday

BREAKFASTS
1. 2-3 *pancakes w/ *syrup or *jelly
   3 slices Canadian bacon
   *scrambled eggs
2. *omelet
   2 slices WW toast w/ 1 tsp. margarine and *jelly (optional)
   2 slices Canadian bacon
3. 4 thin *cinnamon toast
   4 amino acid tablets

A.M. SNACKS
1. 1 cup lite soup
2. 1/2 cup cottage cheese w/ sugar-free fruit

LUNCHES
1. 3-4 oz. lean roast lamb or broiled veal
   1 small potato or *sweet potato
   1 vegetable, cooked or small tossed salad w/ *dressing or 1 cup *slaw
2. 5-6 oz. lean broiled steak
   1 small baked or boiled potato w/ 1 tsp. margarine or 1 tbsp. sour cream
   small tossed salad w/ *dressing or 1 cup *slaw
3. *Chicken Picada
   small tossed salad w/ *dressing

AFTERNOON SNACKS
1. 1/2 bagel w/ 2 tbsp. *Whipped Light Cream Cheese
2. *Waldorf Salad
3. 2 *melba toast w/ 1 tsp. peanut butter on each

DINNERS
1. *Acidophilus Shake
2. 1 thin sliced whole grain toast w/ 2 thin slices Farmer's Cheese, melted
   1 cup soup (optional)
   1/3 cup fat-free yogurt w/ fruit
3.** large tossed salad w/ *dressing
   1 cup soup (optional)
   4 amino acid tablets
4.** 1 bowl vegetable soup
   2 whole grain crackers
   4 amino acid tablets

** (Use #3 or #4 if eating dinner out. "Doggie bag" extra food, if any, for lunch tomorrow.)

P.M. SNACKS
1. 2 fudgesicles
2. 1 piece *Carrot Cake Squares w/ 1 tbsp. *Whipped Light Cream Cheese
3. 3 *melba toast w/ 1/3 slice low-fat cheese on each

* See Recipes

ACTIVITY - WALKING OR MINI TRAMP

WALKING
1. Warm up stroll 4 min.
2. Alternate: <u>10 min</u>. brisk walk, <u>2 min</u>. stroll to total 35 min. Check EHR.
3. Cool down stroll 5 min.
4. Stretch
5. Total time without warm up 40 min.

MINI TRAMP
1. Warm up gentle bounce 4 min.
2. Alternate: <u>10 min</u>. on tramp, <u>2 min.</u> off tramp to total 35 min. Check EHR.
3. Cool down stroll 5 min.
4. Stretch
5. Total time without warm up 40 min.

Goal - 40 min.
Actual Time _____   Goal Reached?_____   EHR? High Low OK

Weekly Success Record
Week #4

*Weight

Weight – Day 22 _____   Total lost this week _____
Weight – Day 29 _____   Total lost to date   _____

* Always weigh yourself first thing in the morning without
   clothes or shoes.

Measurements

Day 22	Day 29	Total lost
chest _____	chest _____	_____
waist _____	waist _____	_____
upper rt. thigh _____	upper rt. thigh _____	_____
upper lt. thigh _____	upper lt. thigh _____	_____
hips _____	hips _____	_____

* Inches lost will be more dramatic than pounds lost when you're
   losing body fat. One pound of fat takes up approximately five
   times the space of one pound of lean!

Activity

Goal – 50 minutes by day 28

Day 22 – Total Time _____   Day 28 – Total Time _____

Water

Day 22 – drank _____ cups		Day 23 – drank _____ cups	
Day 24 – drank _____ cups		Day 25 – drank _____ cups	
Day 26 – drank _____ cups		Day 27 – drank _____ cups	
Day 28 – drank _____ cups			

Energy Level

(Check One)

Day 22 ___Good ___Not Good ___Improving ___Not Improving

Day 23 ___Good ___Not Good ___Improving ___Not Improving

Day 24 ___Good ___Not Good ___Improving ___Not Improving

Day 25 ___Good ___Not Good ___Improving ___Not Improving

Day 26 ___Good ___Not Good ___Improving ___Not Improving

Day 27 ___Good ___Not Good ___Improving ___Not Improving

Day 28 ___Good ___Not Good ___Improving ___Not Improving

* Anytime you are feeling tired for no apparent reason, and/or you are experiencing real hunger in the evenings, you should *increase* complex carbohydrates. First, increase afternoon snacks – whole grain bagel, popcorn, 1/2-1 sandwich on whole grain bread, etc. If tiredness or evening hunger persists, increase food intake at lunch in addition.

Week 4

I. Beginning Weight and Measurements

Weigh yourself in the morning, nude, and record weight on both your Master Success Record, and Weekly Success Record. After recording weight, measure with a snug, not tight, measuring tape and record as indicated on Master Success Record, and Weekly Success Record.

II. Activity Plan

Read over Activity Plan for day 22. If you are not ready to increase as indicated, remain at week 3 level. If you need to increase *more*, add ten minutes to your total time. Be sure to read chapter on stretching.

III. Eating Plan

A. Read over this week's menu and list groceries you need.
B. List recipes you will be using for the week and make sure you include ingredients needed on your grocery list.
C. Make any recipes that you can ahead of time.
D. The word "meat" on menu also includes poultry, fish and seafood
E. Re-read "Weight Loss Special Notes."

Day 22 - Monday

BREAKFASTS
1. 1/2 cup sugar-free cold cereal
   1/2 cup fat-free milk
   1 whole grain toast w/ 2 thin
   slices Farmer's Cheese, melted
2. *hot cereal
   1 WW toast w/ 1 tsp. margarine
   and *jelly (optional)
   4 amino acid tablets
3. 1 English Muffin split w/ 2
   thin slices Farmer's Cheese
   on each
   1/2 cup *yogurt w/ fruit

A.M. SNACKS
1. 1 small piece raw fruit
2. 1/2 cup *yogurt w/ fruit

LUNCHES
1. microwave plate from
   Sunday's dinner
2. 5-6 oz. lean meat
   1 small baked potato or 1 bread
   cooked veggies - small serving
3. 5 oz. lean meat in sandwich
   w/ 2 thin slices WW bread,
   lettuce, tomato, 1 tbsp.
   *mayo (optional)
   1 cup soup or small tossed
   salad w/ *dressing

* See Recipes

AFTERNOON SNACKS
1. 1 small baked potato w/ 1/4
   cup *sour cream
2. *Waldorf Salad
3. 1 whole bagel

DINNERS
1. *Acidophilus Shake
2. 1 cup Lipton's Lite soup -
   appetizer before dinner
   child-sized portions of
   family's dinner foods
3.** small tossed salads - 2
   1st before dinner as appetizer
   2nd with meal (*dressing)
   1 skinless chicken breast
   small serving non seed type
   veggies
4.** bowl of soup
   small tossed salad w/ *dressing
   4 amino acid tablets

** (Use #3 or #4 if eating dinner
    out. "Doggie bag" extra food,
    if any, for lunch tomorrow.)

P.M. SNACKS
1. celery w/ 3 tbsp. *Whipped
   Light Cream Cheese
2. 1/2 small can water packed
   white tuna 1 tbsp. *mayo
   (optional)
3. raw veggies w/ 1/4 cup *onion
   dip

ACTIVITY - WALKING OR MINI TRAMP

WALKING
1. Warm up stroll 4 min.
2. Alternate: 10 min. brisk walk,
   2 min. stroll to total 40 min.
   Check EHR.
3. Cool down stroll 5 min.
4. Stretch (see illustrations)
5. Total time without warm up
   45 min.

MINI TRAMP
1. Warm up gentle bounce 4 min.
2. Alternate: 10 min. on tramp,
   2 min. off tramp to total 40
   min. Check EHR.
3. Cool down stroll 5 min.
4. Stretch (see illustrations)
5. Total time without warm up
   45 min.

Goal - 45 min.
Actual Time _____   Goal Reached? _____   EHR? High Low OK

Day 23 - Tuesday

BREAKFASTS
1. *Acidophilus Shake
   1/2 English Muffin w/ 1 slice
   low-fat cheese, melted
2. 1/2 cup sugar-free cereal
   1/2 cup fat-free milk
   1/2 small banana
   1 thin sliced whole grain
   toast w/ 2 thin slices
   Farmer's Cheese, melted
3. *hot cereal
   1 whole grain toast w/ 1 tsp.
   margarine and *jelly (optional)
   4 amino acid tablets

A.M. SNACKS
1. 1 small piece raw fruit
2. 1/3 cup cottage cheese w/ 1/2
   sugar-free peach half

LUNCHES
1. microwave plate from last
   night's dinner
2. *Beef or *Chicken Stew
   small tossed salad w/
   *dressing or 1 thin sliced
   WW bread
3. 5 oz. lean meat in sandwich
   w/ 2 thin slices WW bread,
   lettuce, tomato, 1 tbsp.
   *mayo (optional)
   1/2 large salt free pretzel
   1 cup soup (optional)

AFTERNOON SNACKS
1. 1/2 sandwich - 1 WW bread
   w/ 1 hard boiled egg white,
   1/2 slice low-fat cheese
2. 1/2 bagel w/ 2 tbsp.
   *Whipped Light Cream Cheese
3. 1/2 cup *rice pudding

DINNERS
1. *Acidophilus Shake
2. *Acidophilus Shake (1/2
   before dinner as appetizer)
   child-sized portions of
   family's dinner foods
3.** small tossed salads - 2
   1st before dinner as
   appetizer
   2nd with meal (*dressing)
   4 oz. fish - broiled or baked
   small serving non seed-type
   veggie
4.** large tossed salad w/ *dressing
   1 cup soup (optional)
   4 amino acid tablets

** (Use #3 or #4 if eating dinner
   out. "Doggie bag" extra food,
   if any, for lunch tomorrow.)

P.M. SNACKS
1. *Acidophilus "Snack" Shake
2. 1/3 cup cottage cheese w/
   *jelly topping
3. raw veggies

*   See Recipes

ACTIVITY - WALKING OR MINI TRAMP

WALKING
1. Warm up stroll 4 min.
2. Alternate: 10 min. brisk walk,
   2 min. stroll to total 40 min.
   Check EHR.
3. Cool down stroll 5 min.
4. Stretch (see illustrations)
5. Total time without warm up
   45 min.

MINI TRAMP
1. Warm up gentle bounce 4 min.
2. Alternate: 10 min. on tramp,
   2 min. off tramp to total 40
   min. Check EHR.
3. Cool down stroll 5 min.
4. Stretch (see illustrations)
5. Total time without warm up
   45 min.

Goal - 45 min.
Actual Time _____   Goal Reached? _____   EHR? High Low OK

Day 24 - Wednesday

BREAKFASTS
1. 4 thin WW *cinnamon toast
   1/2 cup *yogurt w/ Grape Nuts
2. 1 whole grain toast w/ 2 thin
   slices Farmer's Cheese, melted
   1/2 cup fat-free milk
   1/2 cup sugar-free cold
   cereal top w/ sugar-free
   strawberries
3. 1 whole grain toast w/ 1 tsp.
   margarine
   *hot cereal
   4 amino acid tablets

A.M. SNACKS
1. 1 cup lite soup
2. celery w/ 3 tbsp. *Whipped
   Light Cream Cheese

LUNCHES
1. *Beef or *Chicken Stew
   1 thin sliced WW bread
   celery & carrot sticks
2. microwave plate from last
   night's supper
3. 5 oz. lean meat
   1/2 small baked potato w/ 1
   tbsp. sour cream
   1 small serving cooked veggies
   1/2 whole grain bread

*   See Recipes

AFTERNOON SNACKS
1. 1/2 sandwich - 2 tsp. peanut
   butter w/ *jelly (optional)
2. 3 cups fat-free popcorn w/
   Butter Buds powder
3. 1 small baked potato w/ 1
   slice low-fat cheese melted
   on top

DINNERS
1. *Acidophilus Shake
2. 1 cup Lipton's Lite soup
   3 *melba toast w/ 1/3 slice
   low-fat cheese on each -
   appetizer
   child-sized portions of
   family's dinner foods
3.** 1 bowl soup
   2 whole grain crackers
   4 amino acid tablets
4.** 1 cup soup - before dinner
   appetizer
   4 oz. steamed, broiled, or
   baked seafood
   1 small tossed salad w/
   *dressing or non seed-type
   steamed veggies

**   (Use #3 or #4 if eating dinner
      out. "Doggie bag" extra food,
      if any, for lunch tomorrow.)

P.M. SNACKS
1. 1 cup *slaw or raw veggies
2. 1/2 small can water packed
   white tuna, 1 tbsp. *mayo
   (optional)
3. 3 *melba toast

ACTIVITY - WALKING OR MINI TRAMP

WALKING
1. Warm up stroll 4 min.
2. Alternate: <u>10 min.</u> brisk walk,
   <u>2 min.</u> stroll to total 40 min.
   Check EHR.
3. Cool down stroll 5 min.
4. Stretch
5. Total time without warm up
   45 min.

MINI TRAMP
1. Warm up gentle bounce 4 min.
2. Alternate: <u>10 min.</u> on tramp,
   <u>2 min.</u> off tramp to total 40 min.
   Check EHR.
3. Cool down stroll 5 min.
4. Stretch
5. Total time without warm up
   45 min.

Goal - 45 min.
Actual Time _____   Goal Reached? _____   EHR? High Low OK

Day 25 - Thursday

BREAKFASTS

1. 1/2 cup sugar-free cold cereal
   1/2 cup fat-free milk
   1/2 small banana
   1 thin slice whole grain toast
   w/ 1 tsp. margarine
   4 amino acid tablets
2. *hot cereal
   1 whole grain toast w/ 1 tsp.
   margarine & *jelly
   4 amino acid tablets
3. 1 English Muffin w/ 1/2 slice
   low-fat cheese melted on
   each half
   2/3 cup *yogurt w/ fruit

A.M. SNACKS

1. 1 small piece raw fruit
2. 1/3 cup cottage cheese w/
   sugar free fruit

LUNCHES

1. microwave plate from last
   night's dinner
2. 5-6 oz. lean meat
   1 small baked potato w/ 1
   tbsp. sour cream or
   1/3 cup rice
   steamed veggies or small
   tossed salad w/ *dressing
3. 5 oz. lean meat in sandwich
   w/ 2 thin slices WW bread,
   lettuce, tomato, 1 tbsp.
   *mayo (optional)
   1 cup soup

AFTERNOON SNACKS

1. 1/2 bagel w/ 2 tbsp.
   *Whipped Light Cream Cheese
2. 1 whole bagel
3. small baked potato w/ 1 slice
   low-fat cheese

DINNERS

1. *Acidophilus Shake
2. *Acidophilus Shake (1/2 as
   appetizer before dinner)
   child-sized portions of
   family's dinner foods
3.** large tossed salad w/ *dressing
   1 cup soup (optional)
   4 amino acid tablets
4.** 1 cup soup - before dinner
   appetizer
   1 skinless chicken breast or
   4 oz. turkey breast
   1/4 cup rice
   small serving non seed-type
   veggie

** (Use #3 or #4 if eating dinner
   out. "Doggie bag" extra food,
   if any, for lunch tomorrow.)

P.M. SNACKS

1. raw veggies
2. 1 cup Lipton's Lite soup w/ 3
   *melba toast
3. 2 *fudgesicles

* See Recipes

ACTIVITY - WALKING OR MINI TRAMP

WALKING

1. Warm up stroll 4 min.
2. Alternate: <u>10 min.</u> brisk walk,
   <u>2 min.</u> stroll to total 45 min..
   Include 2 EHR checks.
3. Cool down stroll 5 min.
4. Stretch
5. Total time without warm up
   50 min.

MINI TRAMP

1. Warm up gentle bounce 4 min.
2. Alternate: <u>10 min.</u> on tramp,
   <u>2 min.</u> off tramp to total 45
   min. Include 2 EHR checks.
3. Cool down stroll 5 min.
4. Stretch
5. Total time without warm up
   50 min.

Goal - 50 min.
Actual Time _____   Goal Reached? _____   EHR? High Low OK

Day 26 - Friday

BREAKFASTS
1. *Breakfast-In-A-Muffin
2. *hot cereal
   1/2 English Muffin w/ *jelly
   or 1 slice low-fat cheese
   4 amino acid tablets
3. 1/2 cup sugar-free cold cereal
   1/2 cup fat-free milk w/
   peaches or strawberries
   1 WW toast w/
   cinnamon/Equal mixture
   4 amino acid tablets

A.M. SNACKS
1. 1 small piece raw fruit
2. 1/2 cup *yogurt w/ fruit

LUNCHES
1. microwave plate from last
   night's dinner
2. *Beef or *Chicken Stew
   1 thin sliced WW bread
   celery & carrot sticks
3. 5-6 oz. lean meat
   1/2 small baked potato w/ 1
   tbsp. sour cream
   1 small serving cooked veggie
   1/2 whole grain bread (optional)

*   See Recipes

AFTERNOON SNACKS
1. 1/2 sandwich - 1/4 cup *egg
   salad on whole grain bread
2. 1/2 bagel w/ 2 tbsp.
   *Whipped Light Cream Cheese
3. 1/2 cup *rice pudding

DINNERS
1. *Acidophilus Shake
2. 1 cup Lipton's Lite soup
   3 *melba toast w/ 1/3 slice
   low-fat cheese on each -
   appetizer
   child-sized portions of
   family's dinner foods
3.** 4-6 oz. fish or seafood
   1/2 small potato or 1/4 cup rice
   small serving non seed-type
   veggies
   small tossed salad w/ *dressing
4.** large tossed salad w/ *dressing
   1 cup soup (optional)
   4 amino acid tablets

**   (Use #3 or #4 if eating dinner
      out. "Doggie bag" extra food,
      if any, for lunch tomorrow.)

P.M. SNACKS
1. 1 piece *Carrot Cake squares
   w/ 1 tbsp. *Whipped Light
   Cream Cheese
2. 3 *melba toast w/ 1/3 slice
   low-fat cheese on each
3. raw veggies

ACTIVITY - WALKING OR MINI TRAMP

WALKING
1. Warm up stroll 4 min.
2. Alternate: 10 min. brisk walk,
   2 min. stroll to total 45 min..
   Include 2 EHR checks.
3. Cool down stroll 5 min.
4. Stretch
5. Total time without warm up
   50 min.

MINI TRAMP
1. Warm up gentle bounce 4 min.
2. Alternate: 10 min. on tramp,
   2 min. off tramp to total 45
   min. Include 2 EHR checks.
3. Cool down stroll 5 min.
4. Stretch
5. Total time without warm up
   50 min.

Goal - 50 min.
Actual Time _____   Goal Reached? _____   EHR? High Low OK

Day 27 - Saturday

BREAKFASTS
1. 4-5 *pancakes w/ *syrup or *jelly
   3 slices Canadian bacon
   1/2 grapefruit
2. *scrambled eggs or *omelet
   2 slices WW toast (1 tsp. margarine on each)
   2 slices Canadian bacon
3. *bagel breakfast "Danish"
   1/2 grapefruit

A.M. SNACKS
1. 1 cup lite soup
2. 3 *melba toast w/ thin slice Farmer's Cheese on each

LUNCHES
1. large tossed salad w/ *dressing
   1 cup soup (optional)
   4 amino acid tablets
2. chef's salad:
   2 egg whites, 1 1/2 slices low-fat cheese, 3 oz. skinless chicken breast, *dressing or low-fat cottage cheese
3. 4 oz. lean meat in sandwich w/ lettuce, 1 tbsp. *mayo or mustard on 2 thin sliced WW bread
   1 cup soup or small tossed salad w/ *dressing

*   See Recipes

AFTERNOON SNACKS
1. 1/2 sandwich - 1 hard boiled egg white, 1/2 slice low-fat cheese
2. 1 bagel - plain
3. 3 cups fat-free popcorn w/ Butter Buds powder

DINNERS
1. *Acidophilus Shake
2. *Acidophilus Shake (1/2 as appetizer before dinner)
   2 oz. skinless chicken, fish or seafood
   1/3 cup cooked non seed-type veggies
3.** 4-6 oz. skinless chicken, fish or seafood
   small baked potato
   cooked non seed-type veggies or tossed salad w/ *dressing
4.** 1 bowl vegetable soup
   2 whole grain crackers
   4 amino acid tablets

**   (Use #3 or #4 if eating dinner out. "Doggie bag" extra food, if any, for lunch tomorrow.)

P.M. SNACKS
1. celery w/ 3 tbsp. *Whipped Light Cream Cheese
2. 4 *melba toast w/ *jelly
3. 1/4 cup low-fat cottage cheese on 1 sugar-free peach half

ACTIVITY - WALKING OR MINI TRAMP

WALKING
1. Warm up stroll 4 min.
2. Alternate: <u>10 min.</u> brisk walk, <u>2 min.</u> stroll to total 45 min.. Include 2 EHR checks.
3. Cool down stroll 5 min.
4. Stretch (see illustrations)
5. Total time without warm up 50 min.

MINI TRAMP
1. Warm up gentle bounce 4 min.
2. Alternate: <u>10 min.</u> on tramp, <u>2 min.</u> off tramp to total 45 min. Include 2 EHR checks.
3. Cool down stroll 5 min.
4. Stretch (see illustrations)
5. Total time without warm up 50 min.

Goal - 50 min.
Actual Time _____   Goal Reached? _____   EHR? High Low OK

Day 28 - Sunday

BREAKFASTS
1. *Breakfast-In-A-Muffin
2. *scrambled eggs or *omelet
   2 WW toast w/ 1 tsp.
   margarine on each
   2 slices Canadian bacon
3. raisin bagel split w/ 2 tbsp.
   *Whipped Light Cream
   Cheese on each half, topped
   w/ *jelly

A.M. SNACKS
1. 1 cup fresh or sugar-free
   strawberries
2. *yogurt or cottage cheese w/
   fruit

LUNCHES
1. 3 oz. lean baked ham
   small *sweet potato
   2 vegetables and/or tossed
   salad w/ *dressing
2. 4-6 oz. lean broiled steak,
   roast, or skinless poultry
   1 small potato w/ 1 tbsp. sour
   cream or 1/3 cup rice w/ 3
   tbsp. gravy
   1 vegetable and/or tossed
   salad w/ *dressing (small
   serving)
3. spaghetti w/ meat sauce
   small tossed salad w/ *dressing

AFTERNOON SNACKS
1. raw veggies w/ 1/3 cup
   *onion dip
2. 1/2 sandwich w/ 1 WW
   bread and 1/2 slice low-fat
   cheese
3. 1/2 whole grain bagel

DINNERS
1. *Acidophilus Shake
2.** large tossed salad w/ *dressing
   4 amino acid tablets
3. 2 thin sliced WW toast w/ 2
   thin slices Farmer's cheese,
   melted
   1 cup soup
4.** 1 bowl vegetable soup
   2 whole grain crackers
   4 amino acid tablets

** (Use #2 or #4 if eating dinner
   out. "Doggie bag" extra food,
   if any, for lunch tomorrow.)

P.M. SNACKS
1. 1/8 piece *cheesecake
2. 1/2 cup fat-free *yogurt w/
   fruit
3. raw veggies
4. small tossed salad w/
   *dressing

* See Recipes

ACTIVITY - WALKING OR MINI TRAMP

WALKING
1. Warm up stroll 4 min.
2. Alternate: 10 min. brisk walk,
   2 min. stroll to total 45 min..
   Include 2 EHR checks.
3. Cool down stroll 5 min.
4. Stretch (see illustrations)
5. Total time without warm up
   50 min.

MINI TRAMP
1. Warm up gentle bounce 4 min.
2. Alternate: 10 min. on tramp,
   2 min. off tramp to total 45
   min. Include 2 EHR checks.
3. Cool down stroll 5 min.
4. Stretch (see illustrations)
5. Total time without warm up
   50 min.

Goal - 50 min.

Actual Time _____   Goal Reached?_____   EHR? High Low OK

Questions
The Fat To Fit Weight Loss Plan

Why is the first week's Eating Plan different from the three weeks that follow?

The majority of people today eat a light breakfast or none at all, and large evening meals. Evening hunger will halt the most diligent attempt at weight loss. Research studies with people who eat nothing during the day and only one meal in the evening invariably show these people gaining weight. To be successful, any attempt at weight loss must curtail evening hunger at the start – the first week, which is exactly what the first week's Eating Plan is designed to do – end evening hunger. By the fourth or fifth day of the first week with lighter evening eating you will notice that you are getting up in the morning hungry for breakfast. When this happens you will know that you have overcome probably the biggest obstacle to your success with weight control! A healthy breakfast appetite returns only when evening eating is light – a big plus for both health and weight control.

I am concerned about using "Equal" sweetener. Is it really safe?

The FDA Consumer has featured several articles on this product and states that it is the most thoroughly tested food additive ever! It is derived primarily from an amino acid phenylalanine, which occurs naturally in many of our foods. The only problem encountered is with people who are born with a particular genetic disorder who must follow special diets to avoid foods in which this amino acid is found.

After years of extensive testing by the FDA, plus the fact that it is a naturally occurring substance in many of your foods, there is little reason to doubt the safety of this product.

Why do you suggest eating a "snack" before going out to eat? Isn't the afternoon snack adequate?

Usually not. Unfortunately we have a habit of equating "eating out" with "overeating." If you are hungry, the large portions of attractive food set before you, as is the case when you go out to eat, is courting disaster. It is much easier to set aside part of this meal and take it home in a "doggie bag" for tomorrow's lunch, if you're not very hungry when it is served.

My breakfast and lunch are only three and a half hours apart and I am not hungry for a morning snack. On the other hand, my evening meal is more than six hours after lunch and I am usually hungry in the afternoon even with the snack. What should I do?

Adjust your eating to your schedule! Omit the morning snack and have two snacks in the afternoon. Have your morning snack food in the early afternoon and your afternoon snack later in the afternoon. Note the acceptable changes in the two examples of meals and snacks below:

(1)	(2)
Breakfast 8 A.M.	Breakfast 9 A.M.
Lunch 11:30 A.M.	Snack 11:30 A.M.
Snack 2:00 P.M.	Lunch 2:00 P.M.
Snack 4:30 P.M.	Snack 4:30 P.M.
Dinner 7:00 P.M.	Dinner 6:30 P.M.
P.M. Snack as desired	P.M. Snack as desired

I have a problem with evening snacks. I'm fine until I eat my snack, and then I want to continue snacking the rest of the evening. I don't want to discontinue the snack, but what should I do?

You are not alone. Some people have this problem which is usually triggered by previous evening eating habits. Don't despair, there is a "sure-fire" solution. First, choose an evening snack that takes time to eat – the fudgesicles, a dish of raw veggies, etc. Second, postpone your evening snack until right before bed. Do all of your bedtime preparations, relax and unwind while you snack, then immediately brush your teeth and go to bed. This procedure has worked 99% of the time with habitual evening "munchers" who report that looking forward to their bedtime treat helps them avoid eating throughout the evening.

I find that I am getting hungry in the evenings to the point that my stomach is actually "growling." What can I do?

Evening hunger and/or lack of energy results when lunch or afternoon snacks are inadequate. Make sure you are completely satisfied with the amount of food at lunch. Most people on weight loss programs will automatically eat light lunches – a tossed salad or a very "skimpy" sandwich. To judge the lean meat servings suggested for lunch, look at the 4-6 oz. packages of meat at your supermarket, or if you have scales at home, weigh your servings once or twice to help you judge how much you may have. Eat until you are satisfied – don't stuff! Make sure also, that your afternoon snack is adequate. Remember, serving sizes are *suggestions* only! Adjust according to your appetite.

Also, if your lunches and dinners are more than 5 hours apart, you may need to have *two* afternoon snacks – a light one early afternoon and a heavier one late afternoon.

In capsule form, these are the checkpoints for evening hunger and/or decrease in energy:

1. Adequate lunch?
2. Adequate afternoon snacks? Long afternoons may require two snacks – light snacks early afternoon; heavier snacks late afternoon.
3. Make sure evening hunger is really hunger and not habit.
4. See "Weight Loss Special Notes," #23 at the beginning of this chapter.

I know afternoon snacks are important, but once in awhile I get so busy I overlook the time and forget to have one. This doesn't happen often, but when it does, I end up hungry after dinner. What can I do?

The tuna canned in water or chicken breast with melba toast is the best to have in situations like this. It is more filling but very low in fat. You should add some celery sticks on the side for added fiber and to help fill you up.

I have been on the "Fat To Fit" program for two months. I now follow the basics – low fat, low sugar, daily activity, afternoon snacks and light evening eating. Otherwise I have tailored things to suit my schedule and preferences. I am still losing weight, feel terrific but want to know if I will continue to lose to my weight goal with these adjustments?

Absolutely! You are doing exactly what everyone should do and that is to follow the program until you feel comfortable in making changes that you wish, still keeping the basics in mind. Remember the word "SAFE" as explained in the "Maintenance" chapter:

"S" for Sugar intake – keep it low.
"A" for Activity – do it daily until you reach your goal.
"F" for Fat intake – keep it low.
"E" for Evening eating – keep it light.

The first four weeks are designed to help you change your eating habits to the above in a step by step method so you will not be overwhelmed.

I am eating more now than ever before and losing weight. I love it but I don't understand it!

Overweight is seldom due to overeating alone. What you are experiencing is a metabolic increase – you are burning calories and fat faster now which is exactly what is needed to lose weight permanently. A slow metabolism is the cause of overweight and if metabolism is not increased and remains slow, any attempt at weight loss will be only temporary.

Because of the metabolic increase, most people find that even before they reach their weight goal they can eat more than they ever did as an overweight person without a weight gain.

I am absolutely not hungry in the evenings after dinner. Is it necessary to have the P.M. snack?

No. The only absolutely necessary snack is the one in the afternoon. Morning and P.M. snacks are optional, but do have them if you wish.

Is the Acidophilus shake good for small children?

Absolutely! This shake is a very healthy drink for people of all ages. The only change I would suggest is additional carbohydrate for people who need to gain weight. Peak Products, Inc. produces a natural complex carbohydrate powder, "Stamina Plus" which I usually recommend adding to the Acidophilus Shake for thin people or for weight gain.

I don't like milk, and the Tuesday Eating Plan of the first week calls for cereal and milk. Do I have to eat that?

No! You should *never* eat food you don't like! Look at the "Meals and Snacks – Suggestions" and substitute another breakfast.

I am going to a friend's for dinner. She always has fried chicken. What should I do?

First, make sure you have a snack right before you leave or on your way. We can make such good choices when we're not hungry!

Second, pull the skin off the chicken and have veggies as your main dish and the chicken as a side dish.

Third, read question number 1 in the "Living Fit – Twenty Questions" section of the "Special Helps" chapter for a suggestion that has never failed me in situations like this!

I don't see ketchup or mustard on the Eating Plan. May I use these?

Use Heinz Lite Ketchup very sparingly. Regular ketchup has a lot of sugar in it. Mustard is O.K. Once again, it is advisable to read labels.

I get turkey and beef from the "deli." Are these meats good to have?

No! Lunch meats and deli meats are usually high in fat and salt, so eat only occasionally. Get fresh meats and cook your own. I usually cook a turkey breast or other meat on the weekend, slice it in serving sizes and freeze. You'll cut your fat and salt intake, plus save money. Pound for pound, fresh or frozen meats are much cheaper and healthier than pre-cooked meats of any kind.

I don't like salad dressings. Can I use cheese, eggs, croutons, or bacon bits in place of the dressing?

Use the low fat cheese (as recommended in #22 of the "Weight Loss Special Notes" in the beginning of this chapter) egg *whites*, and keep croutons and bacon bits to a minimum.

Can I use already prepared fruit and yogurt mixtures or should I mix my own?

Mix your own. Most yogurt and fruit mixtures have added sugar and those that don't have more flavoring than fruit. Besides, it's cheaper and tastier when you mix your own as directed in the "Recipes" section and takes less than five minutes to mix.

Why do you limit fruit to six small servings weekly and why only in the morning?

Fruit is a very health-promoting food and is very good for you! However, fruit is a combination of complex and simple carbohydrates and women especially do not do as well with weight loss if fruit intake is too high.

Fruit is best in the morning because it is quickly digested and will satisfy hunger only for a short time, and therefore, will not interfere with lunch appetite which should be your most substantial meal of the day.

I am a real non-diet soft drink "freak" and drink six bottles a day. What can I do?

This problem has come up many times. You should cut back gradually. Use the following steps and modify as you feel you can.
1. Cut back the total consumed daily by one.
2. Mix half and half with diet cola, then later begin mixing 2/3 diet with 1/3 regular cola until you are "weaned" to diet cola.
3. Begin cutting back gradually on total consumption of the diet cola.

I don't like mayonnaise on sandwiches. Is it permissible to use margarine?

Yes in teaspoon servings. Try to find a "diet" margarine that will usually have 5 grams of fat per tablespoon as opposed to 11 grams of fat in regular margarine.

Why do you recommend egg *whites* only? What do I do with the yolks?

The egg white is an excellent source of high quality protein (amino acids), and only has a trace of fat. One yolk has 6 grams of fat and 272 milligrams of cholesterol. What should you do with them? The same as you do with the shells that you don't eat–throw them away!

I don't like water! What can I add to it for flavor so I can drink it?

Welcome to the crowd! Many people including myself do not like water. The thing that seems to work best is to put cold water in a quart thermos bottle and sip it throughout the day, gradually increasing your intake to 6-8 cups daily.

Plain water is best without flavoring.

The breads you suggest – why diet and regular both?

1) Whole wheat diet or extra thin sliced:
   Lunch – main dish is protein with side dish carbohydrates. Diet or thin sliced bread has about half the amount of carbohydrates, allowing larger protein consumption.
   Dinner and P.M. Snack – light carbohydrate food needed for decreased energy expenditure at this time of day.

2) Regular whole grain breads:
   Breakfast and Afternoon Snacks – more carbohydrates are needed for energy and to keep blood sugar levels stable at these times of day. Also, afternoon carbohydrates help prevent evening hunger.

I like my baked potato plain. Must I add the margarine or sour cream?

No! Margarine, mayo, Butter Buds, Equal, Sweet 'N Low, etc. are all for flavoring *only*. Omit or adjust any flavoring type of food as desired.

Sometimes in the evenings after dinner, I like to have something to munch on other than my P.M. snack. I'm not really hungry, but my very thin husband and I usually snack and watch television for an hour or so in the evenings, and I'm usually finished with my snack in about 15 minutes. Since I enjoy raw vegetables, could I munch on a few of these in addition to my regular snack?

Yes, you may add raw vegetable snacks in addition to regular snacks anytime you wish.

What do you mean by "fat-free" popcorn?

Popcorn without fat – oil, butter or special cheeses. I have a microwave popping dish to pop regular popcorn that I use. Air popped popcorn is also fat free. Most of the shopping malls have popcorn stands with huge poppers where you can get plain non-fat popcorn.

The one half Acidophilus Shake for dinner appetizer – I usually have mine while I'm fixing dinner for my family, and freeze the other half. The frozen half is always my P.M. snack. Will this cause a problem?

No! I've suggested this many times for the P.M. snack because it not only tastes good but it takes some time to eat, which means it will be more satisfying.

My husband and I went out to eat and I ordered broiled crab cakes. I was shocked when they arrived almost floating in butter! What should you do in a case like this?

Send them back! You are paying the restaurant for two things – service and food prepared the way you want it. Broiled food is ordered by people who want to avoid the fat of frying. Unless the menu stated "broiled in butter," I would be very quick to refuse the crab cakes. Restaurants usually appreciate and will respond quickly to customer preferences but you must let them know what your preferences are.

I am a high school senior. We are not allowed to eat in class, so I can't have my snacks. Will the program work without them?

I know that unfortunately, high school students have split-timed class changes, but what about bath room breaks? Could you have your morning piece of fruit in the restroom on a bathroom break pretense? If not, your afternoon snack is the most important and could be eaten as soon as school ends.

I do know that some high schools have special smoking rooms and if students can manage to get to these, there must be a way to get your snack break, especially your afternoon snack.

Why do you suggest using both Equal and Sweet 'n Low?

Equal leaves no "after taste." The combination is sweeter, more economical and leaves no after taste.

What can I substitute for hot cereal and cottage cheese? I don't like either of these foods.

Cold cereal (sugar-free) may be substituted for hot cereal or a whole grain bread serving. Yogurt may be substituted for cottage cheese.

Be sure to also check "Meals and Snacks – Suggestions" for substitutions.

I don't like following pre-planned menus, and would much prefer planning my own. Is it essential that I follow the four weeks of menus?

It works best if you follow at least the first week and then plan your own meals and snacks if you wish. Read the two chapters "Planning Your Own Menus" and "Quick Weight Loss Plan." However, the day to day Activity Plan included with the menus in this chapter should be closely followed, especially if you are a beginner.

You suggest losing weight at a slower rate, but I am the kind of person who needs the reinforcement of fast weight loss for the first two or three weeks. Can I safely speed up weight loss in the beginning?

Yes. Read the chapter on "Quick Weight Loss" before you begin.

9

PLANNING YOUR OWN MENUS

When you have completed your first four weeks, you may begin planning your own menus based on your food preferences and choices, or you may repeat the previously planned menus from weeks one through four. If you choose to plan your own, this chapter will provide valuable assistance. Whichever you do, make sure you include a variety of foods and that your food choices are not so repetitive that you become bored with eating the same things.

Before beginning week five, if you will be planning part or all of your menus, read both the "Guidelines For Planning Menus," and the "Checklist For Eating Plan," on the following pages. The checklist *must* be used to check each weekly menu at least until you have reached your desired goal. Write down foods on you menu as you wish. Then, upon completion of each week's menu, check your food selections with the checklist. Remember also to record your progress on the Weekly and Master Success Records and include your activity of 50-60 minutes for a minimum of 5-6 days a week until you reach your weight goal.

Included in this chapter you will find "Meals and Snacks – Suggestions," a list of food suggestions for breakfast, lunch, dinner and snacks. These are *suggestions only* and are by no means a complete listing of permitted foods. Favorite foods should not be eliminated! Include these foods, use the checklist and a little common sense and you won't go wrong. For example, if you plan to have Chinese egg rolls plus sweet and sour pork, you obviously will be eating a meal that is high in both fat and sugar. Therefore, this kind of meal would be good to have as a "Binge Day" meal which is explained in the Guidelines. However, if it's Chicken Chow Mein and Egg Drop Soup that you're planning, have regular sized portions for lunch or have smaller portions for dinner.

If the desired food is high in fat and/or sugar, *modify* your intake, do not *omit*! Plan to have the food occasionally at lunch or if an especially rich food, plan it for a "Binge Day."

Following the Guidelines and Checklist you will find the "Overview" which provides at-a-glance food planning in a simplified format. Once you have become familiar with the Guidelines and Checklist, the Overview will provide a quick and convenient reference to assist you with food selections for meals and snacks.

Guidelines For Planning Menus

1. PLAN AHEAD! A planned menu and shopping list is the *only* way to avoid missing snacks, impulsive buying and eating. When planning a full week is next to impossible, then plan at least one day ahead, get your food ready the night before so it will be convenient and ready to have or take with you the next day. This is especially critical if you have a busy schedule.

2. For your menus choose foods either from the previous four weeks menus, "Meals and Snacks Suggestions" and "Recipes" or plan your own. Remember there are many foods that are not listed – choose foods you like and ones that easily fit your schedule so this plan will work for you and become a lifestyle eating habit.

3. Plan the largest meals for breakfast and especially lunch. Up to 10 percent or more of the calories are "lost" through the "thermic effect" of food eaten earlier in the day.

4. Have the most substantial snack in the afternoon. *Never* omit afternoon snacks. These help prevent evening hunger and should become a lifetime habit!

5. You will naturally eat smaller meals when you snack in between. Don't stuff and don't go hungry!

6. KEEP FAT AND SUGAR INTAKE AS LOW AS POSSIBLE! Do not become an obsessive counter of fat grams. There is some fat in almost every food we eat, including fruits and vegetables. Keep your eye on the obvious high fat foods, and from these foods allow approximately 20-25 grams of fat daily while losing weight. Use this number to help guide you when making food choices and when reading nutrition information listed on food labels. Keep in mind also that if sugar is listed as the second or third ingredient on a food label, the food will usually have a high sugar content.

7. Do not have sweets or desserts for at least the first four to six weeks. Use included recipes if you want "sweet" tasting dessert-type foods.

8. Avoid creamed soups. Homemade soups are the best to use whenever possible. After cooking, cool the soup, refrigerate until fat on top is solid and can be removed before eating. Use your own favorite recipes.

9. One "Binge Day" each week may be added (if progress is good) after 4-6 weeks following the guidelines listed below.

   a. Choose one food or one meal for your "Binge."
   b. If you have a dessert food, eat it before 3 P.M., if possible – the earlier, the better.
   c. If you eat a large meal eat it before 5 P.M., the earlier, the better.
   d. After 6 P.M., you are back on your eating plan. If you must have a bedtime snack, choose a very light one.
   e. Binge Day should be included *only* if Eating Plan *and* Activity Plan have been strictly followed all week!
   f. Eat only until satisfied – DON'T STUFF!

10. When menu planning is completed, turn to "Checklist For Eating Plan" and check your menu, making alterations if necessary.

11. Use completed menu to compile your grocery list.

Checklist For Eating Plan

When you plan your own menus, you *must* use this checklist and make necessary changes on *each weekly menu*, based on the checklist where appropriate. Check each item carefully.

1. Have no more than FOUR large or SIX small pieces of fruit per week, and a minimum of ONE of those must be one cup of strawberries or 1 peach. Do *not* count fruit in Acidophilus shakes, cottage cheese/fruit or yogurt/fruit dishes when counting fruit servings.

2. *Evening* meals – must have appetizer before every evening meal unless hunger is absent, or eating "All You Can Eat Salad Bar" (see "Weight Loss Special Notes #21).

3. Four days (minimum), have a tossed salad of some kind for snacks or with a meal.

4. "Seed-type" are starchy vegetables such as corn, peas, lima beans, rice, potatoes, etc. These are best to have at lunch. If eating at dinner, limit to *very small* servings.

5. Supplements – skip 2 consecutive days each week. Write supplements on menu plan as they are to be taken. Have 4 amino acid tablets only with *meals* that do *not* have any or only a very small portion of protein foods such as meats, eggs, cheeses, dairy products, or acidophilus shake. Recommended also – vitamin/mineral supplements plus calcium/magnesium supplements (1500 mg. calcium; 750 mg. magnesium) daily.

6. One *P/F meal a day-limit.

7. One *P/F snack a day-limit.

*P/F = Protein/Fat combination food in which there is a fairly high fat content. Includes all meats, egg yolks, nuts, nut butters and regular dairy products that are *not* fat-free or low-fat. Does not include skinless chicken and turkey, or seafood and fish that is steamed, baked or broiled.

8. Have a *minimum* of four raw vegetable snacks weekly for *evening* or *morning* snacks. The more you choose raw vegetables for *evening* snacks, the better – if you like them.

9. Men may add 2 more grain servings daily (cereals, breads, crackers), and also an additional 2 oz. of meat, fish or poultry, per serving.

10. All visible fat must be removed from meats, and skin from poultry – no frying or breading.

11. If constipation is a problem add 3-4 tbsp. "Quakers Unprocessed Bran" to morning cereal or mix bran with cooked cereal for afternoon snack. This amount may be increased if necessary.

12. Follow "Guidelines For Eating Plan" (#9) for a "Binge Day" food or meal.

Note: You must do your activity plan every day in addition to your eating plan!

An Overview
The Eating Plan Simplified

While most people like to have their menus planned for them, there are others who want only general guidelines and prefer to plan their own. Either way, there are options you may choose from: 1) the four weeks of menus already planned, or 2) those listed in "Meals and Snacks – Suggestions," or 3) use the "Overview" on the following page as a guideline to plan meals and snacks you prefer. When planning menus you may also use a combination of the above which will add even more variety to meals and snacks. Referring to the meals and snacks that are listed will also help make food planning for trips or vacations easy and convenient.

Whatever your choice, it is very important to keep it simple and pleasurable and tailor it to your tastes, needs and schedule to avoid the "dieting mentality." Thinking in terms of being "on a diet," will lead to unnecessary restrictions on food choices and eating accompanied by overly anxious feelings about your "diet." Don't fall into this trap – keep it simple and convenient. If you have a busy schedule, plan your meals to fit easily in your schedule. It is not necessary to plan extra time or special time for snacks, just place them in a convenient place to "munch" on over a period of time, as you work. I like to remind people who claim they don't have time for snacks, of cigarette smokers who always manage time for cigarette breaks no matter how hectic and busy the schedule! I seriously doubt that these people give up smoking for an entire afternoon because there is not enough time, just as I seriously doubt that they ever forgot to take their cigarettes with them. With the unhealthy habit of smoking getting this kind of priority, taking an afternoon snack with you and munching on it as you work deserves at least the same consideration! If afternoon snacks are omitted or forgotten, it is perhaps the priorities that need to be examined and not the busy schedule. The same holds true for activity time.

Choose foods wisely, eat more often, and never "stuff" or go hungry – that's it in a nutshell! Whether you use just the "Overview," or a combination, remember to keep it simple and enjoy!

Breakfast	A.M. Snack	Lunch	Afternoon Snack	Dinner	Evening Snack
MAIN DISH - COMPLEX "CARBS."	**MAIN FOOD COMPLEX "CARBS."**	**MAIN DISH PROTEIN 4-8 OZ.** (low-fat - no frying)	**MAIN FOOD COMPLEX "CARBS."** (from grains, potatoes or rice)	**MAIN DISH COMPLEX "CARBS." FROM VEGGIES**	**MAIN FOOD - COMPLEX "CARBS." AND/OR PROTEIN VERY LIGHT**
• hot cereals • all whole grain breads - bagels, English muffins, etc. • cold cereals - sugar-free • pancakes - whole grain is best, prepare in non-stick pan. • waffles - whole grain, use non-stick spray on waffle iron.	• raw veggies or 1 fresh fruit **OPTIONAL - LOW-FAT PROTEIN** • fat-free yogurt or low-fat cottage cheese w/ fruit, etc.	• lean meat, any kind 4-6 oz. • poultry - skinless 4-6 oz. • seafood 4-8 oz. • fish 4-8 oz. **SIDE DISH COMPLEX "CARBS."** (2-3 small servings from the following) • any veggies - cooked and/or raw • whole grain bread	• bagel - whole grain • popcorn, fat-free • cooked cereal • salt-free pretzels • potato - baked • rice - 2/3 cup • etc. **OPTIONAL PROTEIN/"CARB." COMBINATION**	• any cooked veggies that are <u>not</u> "seed-type" 2-3 small servings • potatoes, rice, <u>small</u> serving (optional) **SIDE DISH - LOW FAT PROTEIN 2-6 OZ.** • lean meat, 1-2 oz. • poultry, skinless, 4 oz. • seafood, 4 oz. • fish, 4 oz.	• raw veggies, **best** "Snack Shake" • 1/2 Acidophilus Shake • yogurt w/ fruit etc. Note: may omit this snack if not hungry after week 1.
SIDE DISH - PROTEIN OR AMINO ACID SUPPLEMENTS • cottage cheese • egg whites • yogurt • etc.	Note: may omit this snack after week 1 if desired.	**OPTIONAL - PASTA** (limit 1x weekly - have small tossed salad on the side.) • spaghetti • pizza • etc.	• 1/2 cup low-fat cottage cheese w/ fruit • 1/2 sandwich • 1/2 bagel with light cream cheese etc.	**APPETIZER** (include unless eating "soup & salad bar") • Acidophilus shake 1/2 • tossed salad, small • 1 cup soup • etc.	
OCCASIONAL - P/F w/ COMPLEX "CARBS." • eggs w/ 1 yolk, Canadian bacon, whole grain toast				**OPTIONAL** Acidophilus shake <u>alone</u> or use 1/2 as appetizer and 1/2 w/ or after dinner or P.M. snack.	

Meals

- A meal should include both "Main Dish" and "Side Dish" unless having a meal listed as "Occasional" or "Optional."
- Use "Appetizer" at dinner as directed.

Snacks

- Have either one "Main Food" choice or one "Optional" choice.
- <u>Never</u> omit afternoon snack.

Meals And Snacks - Suggestions

Breakfasts

1. *Bagel Breakfast "Danish"

2. 1/2 Bagel, toasted w/ 2 tbsp. *Whipped
    Light Cream Cheese
    1/2 cup sugar-free cold cereal
    1/2 cup fat-free milk

3. 1/2 English Muffin w/ 1 tsp. margarine
    *hot cereal (amount desired)
    4 amino acid tablets

4. 1/2 cup fat-free milk
    1/2 cup sugar-free cereal and Equal to sweeten
    (#11 "Weight Loss Special Notes")
    1 whole grain toast with 1 low-fat
    cheese slice melted

5. 2-4 thin whole grain *cinnamon toast
    1/2 cup low-fat cottage cheese w/ unsweetened
    peaches

6. *Egg and cheese muffin

7. *hot cereal
    1 whole grain toast
    1 tsp. margarine
    4 amino acid tablets

8. 1 whole wheat toast w/ 1 slice low-fat cheese,
    melted
    (#22 "Weight Loss Special Notes" — low-fat
    cheese)
    1/2 cup sugar-free cold cereal
    1/2 cup fat-free milk

* See Recipes

9. 2-4 thin *cinnamon toast
1/2 grapefruit
4 amino acid tablets

10. Thin sliced Farmer's Cheese, melted
on 1/2 English Muffin
1/2 cup sugar-free cold cereal
1/2 cup fat-free milk

11. 1/2 bagel w/ 1 tsp. margarine
*hot cereal
4 amino acid tablets

12. 2-4 thin whole grain *cinnamon toast
1/2 cup *yogurt w/ Grape Nuts

P/F 13. 3 eggs (remove 2 yolks) scramble
in non-stick pan
2 whole wheat toast w/ 1 tsp. margarine on each
2 pieces Canadian bacon (optional)

P/F 14. 4-5 pancakes w/ *syrup or *jelly
3 slices Canadian bacon
1/2 grapefruit

P/F 15. *scrambled eggs or *omelet
2 slices whole wheat toast w/ 1 tsp.
margarine on each
2 slices Canadian bacon

16. *Bagel Breakfast "Danish"
1/2 grapefruit

17. 1/2 English Muffin w/ 1 slice low-fat cheese, melted
1/2 cup sugar-free cold cereal w/
1/2 cup fat-free milk

18. *Breakfast-In-A-Muffin

* See Recipes

19. *hot cereal
    1 whole grain toast w/*jelly
    4 amino acid tablets

P/F 20. 2-3 *pancakes w/ *syrup or *jelly
    3 slices Canadian bacon
    *scrambled eggs

P/F 21. *omelet
    2 slices whole wheat toast w/ 1 tsp. margarine and
    *jelly (optional)
    2 slices Canadian bacon

22. 4 thin *cinnamon toast
    4 amino acid tablets

23. 2-4 thin slices *french toast
    *fat-free yogurt with fruit - 1/2 cup or more if desired

24. 1/2 cup sugar-free cold cereal
    1/2 cup fat-free milk
    1/2 small banana
    1 thin slice whole grain toast w/ 1 tsp. margarine
    4 amino acid tablets

25. raisin bagel – split w/ 2 tbsp. *whipped light cream
    cheese on each half, topped w/ *jelly

26. Acidophilus Shake
    1/2 English Muffin w/ 1 slice low-fat cheese, melted

27. 1/2 cup sugar-free cereal
    1/2 cup fat-free milk
    1/2 small banana
    1 thin sliced whole grain toast w/ 2 thin slices
    Farmer's Cheese, melted

* See Recipes

28. 1 whole grain toast w/ *jelly
    1/2 cup sugar-free cold cereal
    1/2 cup fat-free milk
    4 amino acid tablets

29. 1/2 cup sugar-free cold cereal
    1/2 cup fat-free milk w/ peaches or strawberries
    1 whole wheat toast w/ cinnamon/Equal mixture
    4 amino acid tablets

30. 4 thin whole wheat *cinnamon toast
    1/2 cup *yogurt w/ Grape Nuts

31. 1 large raisin bagel – split and toast, spread w/ 2
    tbsp. Philadelphia Light Cream Cheese and sprinkle
    w/ 1 Equal, if desired
    4 amino acid tablets

32. 1 English Muffin w/ 1/2 slice low-fat cheese melted
    on each half
    2/3 cup *yogurt w/ fruit

33. 1 English Muffin w/ 2 thin slices Farmer's Cheese
    on each
    1/2 cup *yogurt w/ fruit

34. raisin bagel split w/ 2 tbsp. *Whipped Light Cream
    Cheese on each half, topped w/ *jelly

35. 1/2 bagel w/ thin slices Farmer's Cheese, melted
    *yogurt w/ fruit

    * See Recipes

A.M. Snacks

1. 1 small piece raw fruit

2. 1/2 cup *fat-free yogurt w/ fruit

3. 1/3 cup low-fat cottage cheese w/ fruit

4. 1 small apple w/ 1 slice low-fat cheese

5. raw veggies – your choice

6. celery w/ 2 tbsp. Philadelphia Light Cream Cheese

7. 1 cup light soup

8. celery w/ 3 tbsp. *Whipped Light Cream Cheese

9. 1 cup sugar-free peaches

10. 2 pieces *melba toast w/ 1/4 slice low-fat cheese on each

11. 1/3 cup cottage cheese w/ peach half

12. 1 cup melon balls

13. 1 cup fresh or sugar-free strawberries

14. 1/2 grapefruit

15. 1/2 small cantaloupe

16. 2/3 cup grapes

* See Recipes

Lunches

P/F 1. 5-6 oz. lean meat
1/3 cup rice or 1 small baked potato w/ 1 tsp.
margarine
cooked veggies

2. 4-6 oz. skinless chicken breast on 2 thin-sliced whole
grain bread w/ lettuce, tomato (1 tbsp. *mayo,
optional)

P/F 3. 5-6 oz. lean broiled steak
1 small baked potato w/ 1 tbsp. sour cream
small *tossed salad (*dressing) or cooked veggies

P/F 4. *tuna melt
small tossed salad w/ *dressing

5. sandwich on 2 thin sliced whole grain bread:
1 slice low-fat cheese, lettuce
1 tbsp. *mayo (optional)
4 hard-boiled egg whites
1 cup soup
carrot and celery strips

P/F 6. 3 oz. lean baked ham
small *sweet potato
2 vegetables and/or tossed salad w/ *dressing

P/F 7. 1/2 cup cooked veggies
small baked potato or *sweet potato, or 1/3 cup rice
4-6 oz. baked or broiled lean meat
1 thin sliced whole wheat bread (optional)

P/F 8. spaghetti w/ meat sauce
small tossed salad with *dressing

* See Recipes

9. large tossed salad w/ dressing
   1 cup soup
   4 amino acid tablets

10. Chef's salad:
    2 egg whites
    1½ slices low-fat cheese
    3 oz. skinless chicken breast
    *dressing (optional)

P/F 11. 4 oz. (lean only) roast beef in sandwich w/ lettuce,
        1 tbsp. *mayo or mustard on 2 thin-sliced whole
        grain bread
        1 cup soup or small tossed salad w/ *dressing

P/F 12. 3-4 oz. lean roast lamb or broiled veal
        1 small potato or *sweet potato
        1 vegetable, cooked or
        small tossed salad w/ dressing or
        1 cup *slaw

P/F 13. 3 oz. lean baked ham
        small *sweet potato
        1 vegetable
        small tossed salad, *dressing

P/F 14. microwave plate from last night's dinner
        (#21 "Weight Loss Special Notes")

P/F 15. 5-6 oz. lean meat
        1/2 small baked potato w/ 1 tbsp. sour cream
        1 small serving cooked veggies
        1/2 whole grain bread

P/F 16. *chili
        raw veggies or tossed salad (*dressing)

* See Recipes

P/F 17.   4-6 oz. lean broiled steak or roast
          1 small potato w/ 1 tbsp. sour cream, or
          1/3 cup rice w/ 3 tbsp. gravy

     18.   1 cup soup
           large tossed salad w/ *dressing
           2 whole wheat crackers or 4 *melba toast
           4 amino acid tablets

P/F 19.   regular pizza 1-2 slices <u>or</u>
          1 whole "Tony's Microlite Pizza"
          (a low-fat pan-size pizza)
          small tossed salad w/ *dressing

     20.   *egg salad w/ lettuce on
           2 thin-sliced whole grain bread
           1 cup soup

P/F 21.   2/3-1 cup *tuna or *chicken salad on lettuce
          w/ 1/2 tomato
          1 large salt-free pretzel

     22.   5-6 oz. poultry or fish
           1 whole grain bread or roll
           cooked veggies

     23.   2/3-1 cup *tuna salad on lettuce w/ 1/2 tomato
           1 large salt-free pretzel
           1 cup soup (optional)

P/F 24.   *turkey or chicken salad (2/3 cup)
             on lettuce with tomato
             2 wasa bread, rice cakes or 3 WW crackers
             1 cup soup (optional)

P/F 25.   2 cups *beef or *chicken stew
          1 thin sliced whole grain bread

      * See Recipes

P/F 26. lean meat (4-6 oz.) on sandwich w/
        thin sliced whole wheat bread, lettuce, tomato
        (1 tbsp. *mayo, optional)

P/F 27. 5-6 oz. lean meat
        1 small baked potato or 1 bread w/ 1 tsp. margarine
        veggies - cooked or raw

     28. large bowl soup (not creamed)
        2 whole wheat crackers
        4 amino acid tablets

P/F 29. lean meat - 4-6 oz.
        small baked potato w/
        1 tsp. margarine or 1 tbsp. sour cream
        *tossed salad or cooked veggies

   * See Recipes

Afternoon Snacks

1. raw veggies w/ 1/3-1/2 cup onion dip

2. small baked potato w/ 1 slice low-fat cheese, melted or 1 tsp. margarine

P/F 3. 1/2 whole grain bagel w/ 2 tsp. peanut butter

4. 3 cups fat-free popcorn w/ Butter Buds powder

5. 3 cups fat-free popcorn w/ 1 tbsp. Parmesan cheese

6. 1/2 sandwich - whole grain bread w/ <u>one of the following</u>:
   1/2 slice low-fat cheese
   1 hard boiled egg white
   1/4 cup *egg salad
   (P/F) 2 tsp. peanut butter
   (*jelly optional)

7. 1/8 slice *cheese cake

P/F 8. small baked potato w/ 1/4 cup *"sour cream"

9. 1 whole grain bagel

10. *Waldorf Salad

11. 1/2 bagel w/ 2-3 tbsp. *Whipped Light Cream Cheese

12. 1/2 cup *rice pudding

P/F 13. 3 *melba toast w/ 1 tsp. peanut butter on each

14. "Oodles of Noodles" cup of instant soup

P/F 15. small apple w/ 1 tbsp. peanut butter

P/F 16. celery (unlimited) w/ 1 tbsp. peanut butter

17. 2/3 cup *hot cereal
   * See Recipes

Dinners

1. *Acidophilus shake

2. *Acidophilus shake (1/2 as appetizer before dinner)
    child-sized portions of family's dinner
    (See #21 "Weight Loss Special Notes")

3. large tossed salad w/ *dressing
    1 cup soup (optional)
    4 amino acid tablets

4. *Acidophilus shake (1/2 as appetizer before dinner)
    1 cup steamed veggies topped w/ 3 thin slices
    Farmer's cheese, melted
    1 whole grain diet or thin sliced bread

5. Acidophilus shake (1/2 as appetizer before dinner)
    2 oz. skinless chicken breast, fish or seafood
    2/3 cup cooked non seed-type veggies

6. Acidophilus shake
    1/2 sandwich on whole grain diet or thin-sliced
    bread w/ 1/2 slice low-fat cheese

7. *Acidophilus shake (1/2 as appetizer before dinner)
    2 oz. lean meat
    1/2 cup cooked or raw veggies
    (meat, veggies optional)

8. *Acidophilus shake (1/2 as appetizer before dinner)
    2 oz. lean meat
    1/2 cup green beans or broccoli
    (meat and veggies optional)

9. *Acidophilus shake (1/2 as appetizer before dinner)
    2-4 oz. turkey or chicken breast
    1/4 cup rice or 1/2 small potato
    1/3 cup kale, green beans, or asparagus

* See Recipes

10. *Acidophilus shake (1/2 as appetizer before dinner)
3-4 oz. broiled fish
1/2 cup cooked green leafy vegetables, green beans,
or broccoli
(meat, veggies optional)

11. 1-2 cups soup ("Weight Loss Special Notes" #17)
2 Wasa w/ 1 thin slice Farmer's cheese on each

12. *tossed salads (2 small):
1st before meal as appetizer
2nd eat w/ meal (*dressing)
4-6 oz. fish or seafood
small serving non seed-type veggies

13. small tossed salads (2 small):
1st before meal as appetizer
2nd eat w/ meal (*dressing)
1 small skinless chicken breast or
2 skinless drumsticks
small serving non seed-type veggies

14. Chef's salad w/ *dressing - use
1 1/2 low-fat cheese slices
plus 3 hard boiled egg whites
2 oz. chicken breast
1 Wasa, rice cake, or 4 *melba

15. Chef's salad: 3 oz. white tuna
1 hard boiled egg white
1 slice low-fat cheese
1/3 cup low-fat cottage cheese
any raw veggies desired

16. 1 cup Lipton's Lite soup - appetizer before dinner
child-sized portions of family's dinner foods.

* See Recipes

17. 1 thin sliced whole grain toast w/ 2 thin slices
    Farmer's cheese, melted
    1 cup soup (optional)
    1/3 cup fat-free *yogurt w/ fruit

18. 4-8 oz. skinless chicken, fish or seafood
    1/2 small baked potato or 1 bread
    cooked non seed-type veggies or
    small tossed salad w/ *dressing

19. large tossed salad w/ *dressing
    4 amino acid tablets

20. 2 thin sliced whole wheat toast w/ 2 thin slices
    Farmer's cheese, melted
    1 cup soup

21. 1 cup soup (not creamed) before meal - appetizer
    4 oz. fish or seafood
    small serving non seed-type veggies
    small tossed salad (optional)

22. 4-8 oz. fish or seafood
    1/2 small baked potato or 1 bread
    small serving non seed-type veggies

23. 2 skinless chicken drumsticks or
    1 small skinless chicken breast
    1/4 cup rice
    small tossed salad w/ *dressing

24. 1/2 small baked potato topped w/ white water-
    packed tuna
    1-2 thin slices Farmer's cheese melted over all
    1/2 cup green beans

25. 1 cup Lipton's Lite Soup
    3 *melba toast w/
    1/3 slice low-fat cheese on each - appetizer
    child-sized portions of family's dinner foods

    * See Recipes

26. 1 bowl soup
    2 whole grain crackers
    4 amino acid tablets

27. 1 thin-sliced whole grain toast w/ 2 thin slices
    Farmer's cheese - melted
    1 cup soup
    small tossed salad w/ *dressing

28. 4-8 oz. fish
    1/2 small potato
    small tossed salad w/ *dressing

29. 4-6 oz. skinless chicken or turkey
    1/2 baked or broiled potato (small)
    1/3 cup cooked non seed-type veggies

30. 1 cup soup
    4 *melba toast w/ 1/4 low-fat cheese slice on each

31. bowl of soup
    small tossed salad w/ *dressing
    4 amino acid tablets

32. 1 bowl vegetable soup
    2 whole grain crackers
    4 amino acid tablets

33. 1 1/2 cup steamed broccoli topped w/
    1 1/2 slices low-fat cheese
    1 whole grain diet bread

    * See Recipes

Evening Snacks

1. *jello - unlimited

2. raw veggies - unlimited

3. 2 *fudgescicles

4. 1/2 sandwich - whole grain diet or thin sliced whole grain bread with <u>one </u>of the following:
     1/2 small can water-packed tuna
P/F 2 tsp. peanut butter
     *jelly
     2 tbsp. *Whipped Lite Cream Cheese
     1/2 slice low-fat cheese
     1-2 oz. poultry breast

5. 1 cup *slaw

6. *Acidophilus "Snack" Shake

7. *Sweet cucumbers

8. 1/2 cup fat-free *yogurt w/ fruit

9. 4 *melba toast w/ *jelly

10. 2 cups fat-free popcorn

11. *jello w/ 1/4 cup cottage cheese

12. raw veggies w/ 1/4 cup *Ranch Dressing or *onion dip

13. 1/8 slice *cheese cake (limit 2x weekly)

14. 1 1/2 cup fat-free popcorn w/ Butter Buds Powder

15. 1/3-1/2 cup low-fat cottage cheese w/ unsweetened peach half

   * See Recipes

16. *Acidophilus Snack Shake

17. 1/2 small can water-packed white tuna w/
    3-4 *melba toast

18. 4 *melba toast w/ *jelly

P/F 19. 2 *melba toast w/ 1 tsp. peanut butter on each

20. 1/3-1/2 cup low-fat cottage cheese w/
    sugar-free strawberries

21. 2 pieces *fudge

22. 1 piece *carrot cake squares
    1 tbsp. *Whipped Light Cream Cheese - optional
    (Limit 2x week)

23. 3 *melba toast w/ 1/3 slice low-fat cheese on each

24. celery w/ 3 tbsp. *Whipped Light Cream Cheese

25. 1/3 cup low-fat cottage cheese w/ *jelly topping

26. 1 cup Lipton's Lite soup w/ 3 *melba toast

27. small tossed salad w/ *dressing

28. 1 large salt-free pretzel

29. 1/4 cup Quaker's Unprocessed Bran w/ 1/4 cup fat-
    free milk
    Equal to sweeten
    (This snack is excellent for constipation)

Note: For additional evening snacks see "Good For You
      Sweets."

* See Recipes

Questions
Planning Your Own Menus

The serving sizes of meals listed - is that raw or cooked weight?

First, let me remind you that serving sizes are suggestions, and you should eat until you feel comfortably satisfied. For example, lunch is primarily a protein meal and if a six-ounce steak is not going to satisfy you, order a larger one. If you find you're satisfied with less, doggie bag the left-overs.

Now, to answer your question, serving sizes suggested are *cooked* weights.

I had chicken breast, a small baked potato, lima beans and a small tossed salad for lunch. I realized I would not be able to eat all the food and was wondering, what would have been the best food to finish and what would have been best to leave?

Since lunch is primarily a protein meal, it is better that you finish the chicken and leave portions of the potato and limas if you are satisfied with less than the entire lunch. These are carbohydrate foods and you will be having a carbohydrate snack later in the afternoon.

I enjoy Chinese and Mexican food occasionally but these are not included in "Meals and Snacks - Suggestions." Are these foods permitted?

Yes, they are permitted. No food is eliminated! Using guidelines in the Overview and the Checklist, you should have no problems including these foods on occasion.

I am the kind of person who would be very content to have all my menus planned for me. Is there any problem staying with the four weeks of menus that are already planned for a long period of time?

This is one of your options. These menus allow a good variety and many choices. As long as you are happy and do not feel restricted in your food choices, you may follow these.

The Sunday menu fits my schedule best on Wednesday this week. Is there a problem with switching these days?

No problem at all to switch an entire day. However, there may be a problem with switching a meal from one day to another and if this is necessary, it is better to switch the entire day.

I have just completed six weeks on this plan and I love it! However, I have purposely not added a "Binge Day" because I tend to get carried away with these kinds of foods. Is the "Binge Day" necessary?

No. If you do not feel comfortable adding a "Binge Day" then don't. Wait until you feel more in control of your food choices and intake. As long as you are not feeling deprived you do not need a "Binge Day."

I like using the "Overview" and planning my own menus. Should I still use the Checklist to check my menus?

Yes, by all means! Using the Checklist will help keep your choices in line with the basics of the program. When you consistently plan menus several weeks in a row that require no changes after checking them with the Checklist, then use the checklist every other week, or once every third or fourth week until you feel your meal planning as suggested in the Checklist has become almost second nature for you.

I found a frozen "light" spaghetti dish that has only 11 grams of fat and is a generous serving. Would this be good to have for lunch?

Yes it would, but also check the protein. Since lunch is a protein meal, if the protein is listed as less than 18 or 20 grams, I suggest you add 1/2 cup of yogurt with fruit or cottage cheese on the side and perhaps carrot and celery strips.

Reading food labels is an excellent practice. You may find many good selections like the above to add variety and convenience to your meals. Food companies are responding to consumer demands with more foods appearing on the market without added sugar and with lower fat content. When checking labels, remember that nutrition information is listed *per serving*, and as such, may be misleading. For example, a nutrition label lists 4 grams of fat *per serving*. Upon checking serving sizes you may find that it would require three times the serving size *listed* to make one *average* serving! This means you must triple the fat grams listed to figure the accurate fat content—12 grams per *average* serving! Some food labels list nutrition information on very small serving sizes of 2 ounces or less. Obviously the fat content will appear lower if listed in these extremely small serving sizes.

I use beef bones with a small amount of beef in my homemade soup. Is this permissible?

Yes. Cool the soup after cooking, refrigerate until fat on top is solid and can be removed before eating. This should be done for any homemade soup to make it fat-free.

Why is an appetizer suggested before evening meals?

Increased hunger results in increased appetite and over-eating usually results. The "appetizers" suggested will actually do the opposite, and dull the appetite so that over-eating is not likely to occur. This practice is suggested specifically to change the habit of eating large evening meals – one of the most notorious fat-producing habits we have!

Interestingly, large evening meals were not always the case, but as our lifestyles changed from rural to urban, the larger meal was eaten in the evening. This has now become a custom (habit) and is one of the primary contributing factors in today's escalating number of weight problems. One of the purposes of this program is to offer alternative choices for evening eating that will satisfy but not fatten.

Avoiding evening hunger is essential. According to Maslow, a behavioral psychologist, hunger is one of the basic, urgent, *determinants* of behavior. As such, it will even influence our food purchasing behavior, which is the reason that most of us prefer not to do our grocery shopping when hungry. The same is true for sitting down to an evening meal, the largest fat producing meal of the day, with hunger determining our food choices. It is much better to have a small amount of food before dinner to reduce hunger, allowing you to be more in control which will result in wiser food choices with little chance of over-eating.

Why should the afternoon snack never be omitted? Do I continue an afternoon snack after I've reached my ideal weight?

Afternoon snacks help prevent evening hunger (see previous question and answer for dangers of evening hunger). They will also increase energy, and yes, they should become part of your eating habits for the rest of your life.

I plan on having an anniversary party. It will also be my "Binge Day," but it will be in the evening after 6 P.M. Will this create a problem?

Not necessarily. Let me remind you that none of the guidelines and not even the checklist is written in stone! Occasional deviations will not cause problems. Don't ever feel that you are "dieting" and cannot occasionally make adjustments to suit the special events of your life. Problems occur when your anniversary type dinner meal is included on a regular basis once or twice *every* week!

If you feel there may be a problem, add an extra activity time the day before and the day after.

Why do you advise skipping vitamin supplements two days a week?

When you have the same thing, day after day, every day, your body tends to "adjust" and the supplements will not be as effective. Skipping two days a week avoids this and they will remain more effective.

The "Binge Day" guidelines state that dessert foods should be eaten before 3 p.m. Our family likes to make homemade ice cream on occasion, but we usually eat it around 4 p.m. Is this too late?

It's not ideal, but one hour will not cause you problems. If you find you're eating the ice cream even later, try to add an extra 30 minutes walking or the mini trampoline later in the evening. It's better to institute some kind of compensation like this than to deprive yourself of something you really enjoy.

When checking my menus with the Checklist, do I include my "Binge Day" meal?

No. The "Binge Day" food is not the normal daily kind of food so do not include it when using the Checklist to check menus. But do follow "Binge Day" guidelines as found in "Guidelines For Planning Menus."

I missed two of my activity sessions this week. Do I omit the "Binge Day?"

Yes. Try to get all of your activity in next week if you wish to add a "Binge Day" meal or food.

I had a smorgasbord with dessert at 1:30 p.m. on my "Binge Day." I was not hungry for the afternoon snack and only slightly hungry that evening and had just a cup of soup. Was it alright to skip the afternoon snack in this case?

You did very well. Sometimes, the problem with omitting afternoon snacks is that you may find yourself very hungry in the evening. Evening eating will add fat to your body very quickly. Since it was your "Binge Day," guideline "d" states, "after 6:00 p.m. you are back on your eating plan." Skipping afternoon snack after a "Binge Day" meal is less likely to find you hungry in the evening, but be aware of the damage evening eating can do, and base your choice on this when having your "Binge Day." On regular days, *never* omit afternoon snacks!

I can't eat my lunch until 2-2:30 p.m. Will this cause a problem?

Not at all. In fact, a later lunch may be a bonus in preventing evening hunger. Adjust snacks so that you are not getting hungry between breakfast and lunch.

I'm having constipation problems. What do you advise?

Quaker's Unprocessed Bran added to morning cereal (3-4 tbsp.). If necessary you may have this amount again in the evening. One way I enjoy bran is to put 1/4 cup in a mug, add a teaspoon of coffee creamer, Equal, a sprinkle of salt and hot water. It tastes like Ralston. I mix it this way for an evening snack occasionally.

The food suggestions listed on the "Overview" – are they the only foods to be used in menu planning?

No! These suggestions are only listed as examples of foods you may use. When reading "P/F w/Complex Carbs.," some people may not understand clearly what that means, so the meal listed will give an example as clarification. The "Meals and Snacks Suggestions," or the previous four weeks of menus or other foods you prefer may be used. Remember – no food is eliminated!

I am absolutely not hungry in the evenings, which surprises me because I was always an "evening eater"! Since I am not hungry, must I have the appetizer?

Use your discretion and have the appetizer when you feel you need help with controlling evening appetite. If you don't feel you need it, don't use it. If you find you are eating more than you should for dinner, have the appetizer to dull your appetite and help modify your food intake. Each person is different and needs to make adjustments necessary to their own unique needs!

I really don't have the time to make all of the recipes, so I make only those I really like. For example, I have always liked tuna and chicken salad without the mayonnaise, and prefer the baked potato plain without "sour cream." I would like to know if these adjustments can be made to suit my taste?

Absolutely! Equal, cinnamon, mayonnaise, Butter Buds, margarine, salt and many other ingredients are included for *taste* only and have no other value. Omit any of these things whenever you wish!

Your recipes are excellent! The jelly tastes so good that my family actually prefers it to real jelly. Are you planning on writing a recipe book with more of these delicious recipes?

As a matter of fact, I am. The recipe book will be my next book and has already been started.

I am pleased that you are introducing your family to the foods included in your eating plan. The entire family will benefit, and it is a much better way to express your love for them than baking cakes, cookies and pies!

When I have a birthday, I will invariably receive a box of candy and a birthday cake. How should I handle this?

These kinds of gifts are given by people who do not understand their potential health hazards. Accept them graciously, but once they are given to you they are yours to do with as you choose. Your choice will be whether to throw away (*waste*) or eat (*waist*) – which do you want? If it is very difficult for you to throw away food, you may consider freezing, and eating on occasion for a "Binge Day" food, but if you are the kind of person who will eat frozen cake as quickly as unfrozen cake, base your choice on this! One husband and wife I know did not begin losing weight until their supply of "junk food," which they didn't want to throw away, was gone. Then they began losing weight, and having learned a lesson, decided never to keep that kind of food on hand again!

Food for thought – if you had some medication on hand after your doctor discontinued it, would you take it anyway to avoid "wasting" it?

There are two social events that I must attend this week, both of which look like "Binge" days. What would you suggest?

In any situation like this it is very important to *plan ahead* and *compensate*. Here are some suggestions:

- Follow the Quick Weight Loss plan for several days prior to these events or plan one extra activity time the day before and the day after *each* event, or . . .
- Modify food intake at one or the other event so that you will have only one "Binge" day.
- Be sure to have something to eat right before you leave home or on the way to the event to dull your appetite and keep you in control.

10

QUICK WEIGHT LOSS PLAN

To Remedy Occasional Overindulgences

The "Quick Weight Loss" is an excellent plan for temporary use after an occasional "slip" or overindulgence to avoid weight gain and get you back on track. It has recently been expanded to serve also as an effective method for those who wish to lose weight faster, although I do not totally support a fast weight loss approach. Let me explain.

The primary goal of the "Fat To Fit" program is to change some of your habits to those that will increase metabolism which, in turn, will produce a natural and permanent normalization of weight without dieting. With metabolic increases, the body uses fat more rapidly which results in a more dramatic loss of inches than pounds. For example, when *eight* pounds of fat are lost, inches lost will be approximately the same as if losing *fourteen* or more pounds through a dieting approach. The reason—body fat is light in *weight* but takes up pound for pound, *five* times the space of lean tissue! Dieting produces a greater loss of the heavier lean tissue which equates to more pounds lost, but fewer inches lost. Your body will get smaller, quicker, if the pounds you lose are body fat.

While this concept is easily understood, there are still some people who are not content to lose pounds slowly and begin cutting calories to lose weight faster. Needless to say, cutting calories compounds their weight problems, and in a very short time, metabolic decreases will halt their weight loss.

For Fast Weight Loss

It became evident that there would always be a few who would insist on losing faster with this no-win approach unless an alternative was offered. Therefore, for those who need the motivational "boost" of fast weight loss for just the beginning weeks, as well as those who have been indoctrinated with the fast weight loss dieting concept, the "Quick Weight Loss" was expanded to provide fast weight loss without a metabolic decrease.

I highly recommend the "Quick Weight Loss" as excellent to remedy a "slip," however I must emphasize that I include it as a fast weight loss plan with reservation. While it is the only way to speed up weight loss without causing a metabolic decrease, and is perfectly safe, be aware that it is more demanding and as such, when used for an extended period of time, may lead to discouragement. If this happens, return immediately to the regular program keeping in mind that a slower weight loss is not only easier but will allow time for the development of new habits to make the weight loss permanent. If you lose only one pound a week you will be 52 pounds lighter next year at this time. A year is going to pass when a year passes and you will either be thinner or not. Why rush?

If you wish a faster weight loss, it is recommended that you follow the menu for Week #1 of the regular plan and then begin the "Quick Weight Loss" program. Some people, needing the motivation of a fast loss at the beginning, follow the first week's regular menu, then the "Quick Weight Loss" to give them a quick beginning loss of 15 or 20 pounds. With that incentive under their belts, they switch to the regular program to continue their weight loss at a slower pace. Whichever you prefer, the "Quick Weight Loss" program calls for strict adherence to *both* Eating and Activity plans. Do *not* attempt the Eating Plan without the Activity Plan or you may institute a metabolic decrease!

A word of warning—the "Quick Weight Loss" is not intended for those who are severely overweight or for those whose medical problems require a very slow beginning period for the activity.

Guidelines For Quick Weight Loss
(Never use Eating Plan without Activity Plan!)

I. **Eating Plan:**

    A. Must eat 3 meals and 3 snacks daily. Use only "Meals and Snacks Suggestions" for breakfast, lunch and afternoon snacks.

    B. *All* evening snacks – raw veggies only.

    C. *All* morning snacks – a small piece raw fruit only.

    D. *All* evening meals – alternate choices below:

        1. Acidophilus shake – *alone*, or with #2 or #3.

        2. Vegetables – 1 cup (do *not* include "seed-type" vegetables, rice or potatoes).
           Lean skinless poultry or fish – 2 oz.

        3. Large tossed salad w/ dressing as listed in recipes.

        4. 4-8 oz. skinless poultry or seafood (*not fried*), 1/2 cup veggies cooked and/or raw, small baked potato or 1 bread. (Limit this dinner to *once* per week.)

    E. Read "Weight Loss Special Notes" before planning menus.

II *Activity Plan* – 80-90 minutes daily (Choose A or B):

    A. 40 minute fast walk or mini-tramp *two* times every day at exercise heart rate:

        1. Before breakfast

        2. Before or after lunch or afternoon

        3. Before or after evening meal

    B. Fast walk or mini-tramp *two* times every day at exercise heart rate:

        1. 60 minutes A.M. + 30 minutes P.M.

           or

        2. 30 minutes A.M. + 60 minutes P.M.

* Follow Activity guidelines, beginning and increasing at your own pace! Do not *begin* at times listed above if you are a beginner. Check exercise heart rate chart.

How To Use Quick Weight Loss

I. For faster weight loss follow a) or b):

    a) Use menu for Week One and then begin using "Quick Weight Loss." Be sure to adjust Activity Plan of "Quick Weight Loss" to your level if you are a beginner.

    b) Use "Quick Weight Loss" Monday through Wednesday, then use regular menus or the Overview for meals and snacks Thursday through Sunday each week.

II. For a "Repair Kit" when overindulging occurs while losing or maintaining follow a), b), or c):

    a) Use "Quick Weight Loss" two or three days after an unplanned overindulgence.

    b) Use one week before and one week after vacations or extended holidays.

    c) Use one day before and one day after a big eating event – party, banquet, etc.

Planning Your Own Quick Weight Loss Menu

Breakfast: "Meals and Snacks Suggestions" – your choice (pp. 167-70)

A.M. Snack: 1 small piece raw fruit

Lunch: "Meals and Snacks Suggestions" – your choice (pp. 172-75)

Afternoon Snack: "Meals and Snacks Suggestions" – your choice (p. 176)

Dinner: Any *one* of choices below:
1. Acidophilus Shake
2. Acidophilus Shake (1/2 as appetizer)
   vegetables - 1 cup (avoid "seed type," rice and potatoes)
   2 oz. lean skinless poultry or fish
3. Acidophilus Shake (1/2 as appetizer) - optional
   large tossed salad w/ dressing as listed in recipes (top w/ 1 slice
   low-fat cheese and 2 cooked egg whites - optional)
4. 4-8 oz. skinless poultry or seafood (not fried)
   1/2 cup veggies, cooked
   small tossed salad or raw veggies of your choice
   small baked potato or 1 diet bread
   (Limit this dinner to once a week)

Evening Snack: Raw veggies as desired

Activity Plan: 80-90 minutes daily – see "Guidelines For Quick-
   Weight Loss" (p. 195)

Questions
Quick Weight Loss

If quick weight loss slows metabolism, how will this approach work?

The activity as listed will prevent the metabolic slow down. It is for this reason that the Eating Plan should never be attempted without the Activity Plan!

Could I follow the weekly menus as written and make the changes as suggested on the "Quick Weight Loss" chart or must I plan my own?

You can do either, but if you plan your own, you must use only breakfast, lunch, and afternoon snacks as listed in "Meals and Snacks Suggestions."

Why is it necessary to read the "Weight Loss Special Notes?"

You must know what kinds of cheeses, breads, cereals, etc. to use. There is other information you need to know also. These should be read at least once weekly for the first four to six weeks.

Do I still plan a weekly menu?

Yes! Forgotten snacks and missed meals are the result of not planning and will halt weight loss very quickly.

How fast will I lose on the "Quick Weight Loss" program?

That is difficult to answer. It depends to a large degree upon how quickly you are able to increase your activity time, and how strictly you follow the guidelines. Weight loss will vary from week to week with beginning weight loss always greater. The more overweight you are, the more quickly you will lose, especially in the beginning weeks. Women of 215-240 pounds have reached normal weight within 5-6 months on the "Quick Weight Loss" program, and men usually lose a little faster.

Does the weight stay off?

Yes, if you go immediately to the maintenance program which will be a real treat after the rigidity of the "Quick Weight Loss" program.

Do many people use the "Quick Weight Loss" as opposed to the regular program?

Most people who use "Quick Weight Loss," follow the first week's menu and then the "Quick Weight Loss" for two or three weeks for extra motivation that fast weight loss gives. Usually they opt into the regular program after this. However, those who have stayed with the "Quick Weight Loss" have usually been very goal oriented, highly motivated and determined people.

Is the "Quick Weight Loss" nutritionally sound?

Yes, especially if vitamin/mineral supplements are included. It is high in fiber and complex carbohydrates, moderate in protein and low in fat and sugars.

Can I still use 1/2 the Acidophilus as an appetizer and the other 1/2 as dinner dessert with the #2 evening meal on the "Quick Weight Loss" plan?

Yes, by all means. You may also have 1/2 for an appetizer before dinner #1 or dinner #2 and have the other 1/2 for the P.M. snack plus some raw veggies.

What about breakfasts, lunches and afternoon snacks? The guidelines do not mention them.

Under "I. - The Eating Plan," letter "a", you are instructed to use only "Meals and Snacks Suggestions." This means breakfasts, lunches and afternoon snacks are to be selected from these suggestions only.

If I want to have only the Acidophilus shake for all my evening meals, must I alternate the other selections?

It is best to alternate at least one of these choices to prevent boredom and for better nutrition. The Acidophilus shake is an excellent choice at approximately 30 grams of protein and practically no fat, but usually if you have a food so often that you get tired of it, you may not want it again for months.

What kind of vegetables are "seed-type"?

You are instructed to read "Weight Loss Special Notes" where you will find an explanation along with other valuable information you will need. "Seed-type" vegetables are those that are seeds – beans, corn, peas, etc.

I want to do Activity Plan "A." I have time before breakfast and in the afternoon, but not in the evening. How can I arrange my activity?

The Activity Plan states 80-90 minutes daily. Since you only have two available times, divide your time and do part of total time in the morning and the other part in the afternoon. The important point here is to have at least two different times for your activity, with the total time 80-90 minutes every day.

I am just beginning my activity and I get too tired to do more than 20 minutes of the activity twice a day. What can I do?

This is one of the limitations of the "Quick Weight Loss." Do not force the activity! Continue at no more than your 20 minute pace until you can comfortably increase. Make *sure* you follow guidelines for beginning your activity!

If the "Quick Weight Loss" is nutritionally sound, increases metabolism and produces a faster weight loss, why do you hesitate to recommend it?

Adherence is much more difficult and therefore it is much more likely to discourage those who are looking for a permanent end to weight problems. Changing eating and activity habits is more effective if done slowly in a step by step process. Also, people who are twenty or more pounds overweight should add a resistance exercise program to prevent a "flabby" appearance that will often accompany fast weight loss. While it is quick, it does require a much larger daily expenditure of time to be done effectively.

I went to a party last night and the food was so good I really got carried away. How long should I stay on the "Quick Weight Loss" to "undo" the damage?

This depends upon how much you ate of what. If the foods you overate were desserts, you ate foods high in both fat and sugar which is probably the worst combination of all for weight gain.

A day or two is usually adequate, but only you know how much you overindulged. You may want to opt for two, three, or four days based on your motivation and overindulgence.

Whatever you do, avoid guilt feelings as much as possible! There is not a person alive who has not, at some time, overindulged – it's part of our human nature. Recreate the situation mentally and "walk" yourself through it to see if you can discover some alternatives you might want to use the next time. In this manner, your "mistake" can be turned into a valuable learning situation that can be used in similar situations in the future!

I am going on a cruise and I plan to enjoy the food – perhaps overindulging at times if I feel so inclined. Could I use the "Quick Weight Loss" for a week before I go and then a week after I come back?

Good thinking! Yes, do exactly that and you'll be fine. It's always a good idea whenever possible to use this approach both before and after to give the metabolism an added "nudge." This kind of compensation is excellent in tailoring your lifestyle so that you are never deprived and can enjoy any of the foods and events you wish.

11

RECIPES

ACIDOPHILUS SHAKES

Acidophilus Shake

1/3 cup water

1/4 tsp. pure vanilla extract

4 packets Equal sweetener plus
   1 Sweet 'n Low (adjust as desired)

1/4 cup Colombo Fat-Free Yogurt

3 tbsp. 100% Egg Protein Powder

8-9 ice cubes

Add <u>one</u> of the following to above ingredients:

- Strawberry - 1 tbsp. *Strawberry Extract and 5-8 strawberries (unsweetened)
- Cherry - 1 tbsp. *Cherry Extract and 4-6 cherries (unsweetened)
- Blueberry - 1/2 cup Blueberries (unsweetened)
- Banana - 1/2 frozen Banana
- Butter Nut - 1 tbsp. "Vanilla Butter & Nut Extract"

Blend in blender.

*McCormick's Extracts recommended.

Chocolate or Vanilla Acidophilus

2 tbsp. Colombo Fat-Free yogurt and water
2/3 cup water
1 1/2 pkg. Alba High Calcium Shake- chocolate or vanilla
1/4 tsp. pure vanilla extract
3 Equal
1 Sweet 'N low
2 tbsp. (rounded) 100% Egg Protein Powder
8 ice cubes

Blend in blender.

Acidophilus "Snack" Shake
(For Evening Snacks)

2/3 cup water
2 tbsp. Colombo Fat-Free Yogurt
1/4 tsp. pure vanilla extract
1 tbsp. 100% Egg Protein Powder

4 Equal
1 Sweet 'N Low
8-9 ice cubes

Add <u>one</u> of the following:

- Strawberry - 1 tbsp. strawberry extract and 5 strawberries (sugar-free)
- Cherry - 1 tbsp. cherry extract and 4 cherries (sugar-free)
- Blueberry - 1/3 cup blueberries (sugar-free)
- Banana - 1/2 small banana
- Butternut - 1 tbsp. "Vanilla Butter and Nut" extract

*Acidophilus Shake
Time Saver Breakfast

A. Mix all ingredients except ice and blend.
B. Put blender with ingredients in refrigerator overnight.
C. Next morning, add ice cubes, mix and drink on your way to work.

*Be sure to include whole grain toast or other carbohydrate food when having Acidophilus for breakfast.

BREAKFAST FOODS

Bagel Breakfast "Danish"

1 raisin bagel - split in half
2/3 cup cottage cheese (1/3 cup on each half)

Put in microwave or toaster oven and heat until cottage cheese is hot.
Remove and sprinkle with cinnamon and Equal.

Breakfast Eggs or Omelet, Low-Fat

Scramble 1 whole egg and 2 egg whites or 3 egg whites with 1 drop
yellow food coloring added. You won't know the yolks are missing!
You can also make a delicious omelet with 3-4 egg whites and two drops
of yellow food coloring. Add onions, green peppers, 1 tbsp. of ham or 2 slices
Canadian bacon bits (optional) or any other vegetables you like.
Melt 1 slice of low-fat cheese on top after cooking in non-stick pan. If
you use the cheese you won't need salt!

Breakfast-In-A-Muffin

1 English Muffin, toasted w/ 1 slice low-fat cheese melted on bottom half.
Top with 2 sliced hard boiled egg <u>whites</u> and 2 slices Canadian bacon.

Cinnamon Toast

2 slices toasted whole wheat bread.
Slice through middle to make 4 thin slices.
Put 1 tsp. Butter Buds <u>mixture</u> on each slice or 1/2 tsp. Corn Oil Margarine
on each. Sprinkle with Equal and cinnamon mixture.
(Use 1/2 recipe for evening snack)

French Toast

Toast 2 slices whole wheat bread – cool.
Slice through middle to make 4 thin slices. Set aside and mix the following:

2 eggs - beaten (remove 1 yolk)	sprinkle salt
1/4 tsp. cinnamon	1 tbsp. milk – fat-free

Dip each slice of thin toast and "fry" in non-stick pan. Immediately after removing from pan, spread 1/2 tsp. margarine or Butter Buds mixture and sprinkle Equal sweetener on each slice.

*Hot Cereal

1/2 cup long cooking oatmeal or 1/3 c. oat bran
2 rounded tsp. Butter Buds powder
1 Sweet 'N Low
2 Equal

Put all of above ingredients in a large mug or bowl. Pour boiling water over all and mix. Let stand a minute or two while you fix your toast. Stir and serve. If consistency is too thick, add more hot water. Adjust sweetness as you wish.
*Any hot cereal may be used, but all others must be cooked first. Do not use instant cereals!

Whole Grain Pancakes

1 1/2 c. flour	1/4 c. bran
1 1/4 c. whole wheat flour	1/4 c. oatmeal
1/2 c. corn meal	2 1/2 tbsp. baking powder
1/4 c. wheat germ	1 1/2 tsp. salt

Mix ingredients and store in tightly closed container in refrigerator.

To make pancakes:

1 1/2 c. fat-free milk	1 c. low-fat cottage cheese
3 egg whites	3 c. mix (above)

Blend cottage cheese and 1/2 c. of the milk. Combine cottage cheese/milk mixture with the remainder of the milk and egg whites. Add to pancake mix. Stir just until mixed. Bake on non-stick 400 degree griddle or in non-stick fry pan. Yield: 12 pancakes (3 inch). 4-7 pancakes = 1 serving. Serve with jelly (see recipe) or maple syrup recipe below. Freeze left over pancakes, or use for "Strawberry Short Cake" recipe. Frozen pancakes may be reheated in toaster or microwave as needed.

Maple Syrup

Mix 2 Equal with 2 tbsp. water. Add 2 tbsp. real maple syrup and mix well. Yield: 1 serving.

Butter Buds Mixture

1 packet of Butter Buds.
Safflower oil (substitute for water in recipe on Butter Buds package).
Stir well and keep refrigerated.
Use in same serving sizes as recommended for margarine.

LUNCH AND DINNER DISHES

Egg Salad

4 hard boiled egg <u>whites</u>
1/2 of 1 egg yolk
2 tsp. dehydrated onion flakes
1 drop yellow food coloring
2 tsp. water

1/4 tsp. Butter Buds powder
2 tbsp. *"mayo" (see recipe)
sprinkle of salt to taste

Chop egg whites. Mash 1/2 egg yolk and mix with the rest of ingredients. Recipe = 1 serving for lunch. Omit salt when using in sandwich with low-fat cheese slice.

Chicken or Turkey Salad

Use "mayo" (see recipe) <u>only enough to hold mixings together</u>. May add egg whites, onions, and parsley if desired. An occasional already prepared salad when eating out is permissible.

"Mayo"

1 c. light mayonnaise
1 c. low-fat cottage cheese
1/4 c. water

Blend cottage cheese and water in blender until smooth. Pour into bowl and mix with the mayonnaise. Put mixture in an empty mayonnaise jar and fool your family!

Tuna Salad

Mix water packed tuna, finely diced onions, egg whites, parsley and low-fat cottage cheese. Good!

If you like sweet pickle in your tuna salad, make the recipe for sweet cucumbers, let stand in refrigerator for 3 or 4 days and use in place of sweet pickle.

Baked Potato "Meal"

Bake a small potato; scoop out potato and fill potato skins with cooked veggies (1/2 - 1 c.).
Place 1 slice low-fat cheese on top and melt over all. Good for dinners.

Beef Stew

2 lbs. round roast	1 tsp. salt (and pepper if desired)
2 medium potatoes	2 extra large onions - diced
2 small frozen pkgs. peas & carrots	1 tbsp. Worcestershire Sauce

Cut round roast into cubes. Remove all visible fat. Brown and drain on paper towels. Put back into pan and add worcestershire sauce. Simmer 3 minutes. Add diced onions and simmer slowly while peeling and cutting potatoes in cubes. When onions are tender, add salt and pepper, potatoes, peas and carrots, and just enough water to barely cover ingredients. Simmer slowly 1 hour.
2-2 1/2 c. = lunch serving; 1 c. = dinner serving.

Chicken Picada

1/2 c. cooked rice
1 extra large or 2 medium pieces of chicken breast, cooked and skinned
1 tbsp. lemon juice
1-2 tsp. Butter Buds Powder
1/2 pkg. "Trim" Chicken Soup mixed with 1/2 c. water

Dice chicken, put over rice, sprinkle on Butter Buds, lemon juice and soup mix. Heat until hot in microwave or toaster oven. Serves 1 for lunch. Reduce rice to 1/4 c., use 1 small chicken breast and add small tossed salad or green beans on the side for dinner.

Candied Sweet Potatoes

Sprinkle Butter Buds powder and cinnamon on sweet potatoes, cook and before serving sprinkle w/ Equal.

Chicken Stew

3½ lbs. chicken	1 tsp. paprika
2 medium potatoes	1 extra large onion
2 small pkgs. frozen corn	2 tsp. parsley
1 tsp. salt and pepper	

Steam chicken and remove all skin and fat. Cool chicken stock in freezer to reach a cold temperature quickly. Bone and refrigerate chicken. Peel and cut potatoes and onions into cubes. When chicken stock is cold, remove all solidified fat from top. Add extra water if necessary and cook onions and chicken until onions are tender. Add paprika, parsley, salt and pepper. Simmer 15 minutes. Add potatoes and corn. Simmer slowly 1 hour.

2-2½ c. = lunch serving; 1 c. = dinner serving

Crispy "Fried" Chicken

2/3 c. non-fat dry milk	salt and pepper (optional)
3½ tsp. paprika	chicken breasts or cut up fryer 3-3½ lbs.

Wash chicken, remove skin and all visible fat. Lightly salt and pepper if desired. Mix dry milk and paprika and thoroughly coat each chicken piece in the mixture. Place in large shallow pan that is non-stick or use a non-stick cooking spray. Bake 30-40 minutes per pound in 350 degree oven until well done and crispy brown.

Deluxe Crispy Fried Chicken

Double the dry milk and paprika above, place in large food-storage plastic bag and mix well. Wash and remove skin and all fat from chicken. Lightly salt and pepper if desired. Drop 2 pieces at a time into bag with dry milk mixture and shake to lightly coat chicken pieces. Shake off excess. Mix well 1 whole egg, 1 egg white and 1/2 c. water in large bowl and dip coated chicken pieces in mixture, one piece at a time. Put back into bag with milk mixture again and coat well. Bake 350 degrees in large shallow, non-stick pan for 30-40 minutes per pound until well done and crispy brown.

Chili

2 lbs. ground round beef	2 extra large onions - diced
2 large cans kidney beans	1 tsp. salt
3 tbsp. chili powder	1 tsp. fructose
2 large cans tomatos	

Cook ground round and sliced onions until meat is brown. Add rest of ingredients. Let come to a boil, turn on low heat and simmer 2 hours. Cool, refrigerate and remove fat from top before serving. May freeze leftovers. 2 c. = lunch serving; 1 c. = dinner serving.

Egg Sandwich

2 slices toasted whole wheat bread
3 hard boiled eggs
1 slice Country Singles cheese

Melt cheese on toast. Cut eggs in half, remove yolks and discard. Place whites, cut side down on cheese toast. Needs no salt!

Home-Made Soups

Make your own favorite soup recipe. Cool and put in refrigerator until cold and fat on top is solid. Remove all fat before serving. You may want to put in containers and freeze.

Salmon Cakes

1 151/2 oz. can of salmon, drained	2 tbsp. non-fat milk powder
1 egg white	3 tbsp. bread crumbs
2 tbsp. dehydrated onion flakes	1 tsp. lemon juice
11/2 tsp. dried parsley	

Beat egg and add onion flakes, parsley, milk and lemon juice. Stir and add to drained salmon. Mix well. Add bread crumbs – just enough to hold the mixture together. Pat into 4 patties and cook in non-stick skillet for about 15 minutes on medium heat. Turn half way through. Do not let them get too brown. 2 patties for lunch, 1 patty for dinner.

Slaw

Shredded cabbage (add some grated carrots if desired)
Blend low-fat cottage cheese in blender and add vinegar and Equal to taste
for dressing. Mix and refrigerate 1 hour before eating.
1 c. = P.M. (evening) snack or may eat w/ evening meal.

Broccoli - Cheese Casserole

1 c. rice
1 c. fresh, chopped or canned mushrooms, drained
1 pkg. chopped broccoli
1 tbsp. corn starch
Farmer's Cheese Slices
2-3 tbsp. dehydrated onion flakes
2 tsp. Butter Buds Powder

Cook broccoli and rice. Drain both. Save and cool 1/2 c. liquid from broccoli.
Mix Butter Buds and corn starch and add to cooled 1/2 c. broccoli liquid.
Mix and simmer until thickened. Mix all ingredients except cheese and
simmer 10 minutes. Top with cheese and heat until cheese melts.

"French Fries"

1 medium-small Irish potato
1 tsp. Safflower oil
paprika

Preheat oven to 475° F. Scrub potato, but do not peel. Cut into strips and
dry well with paper towels. Toss in a bowl with oil. Spread in single layer
on cookie sheet, dust very lightly with paprika and place in preheated oven
for 35 minutes. Crisp and brown by placing under broiler for 1-2 minutes.
Makes 1 serving.

Tuna Melt

1/3 c. tuna salad or plain water packed tuna
1 or 2 slices tomato with generous sprinkle of Italian Seasoning on top
2 thin wedges of Farmer's Cheese slices on top

Broil or microwave until cheese melts thoroughly. Place on lettuce leaves and serve on toasted whole wheat bread or English Muffin.

Turkey Cutlets

1/4 c. flour   1 lb. turkey cutlets from breast
1/4 c. oat-bran   2 egg whites

Mix flour and oat-bran. Lightly salt, then dip turkey cutlets into egg whites. One at a time, place cutlets into the oat-bran mixture, coating each well. In a non-stick pan, fry until golden brown. Makes 2-3 servings for lunch; 4 servings for dinner.

"Sour Cream"

Blend 1/3 c. cottage cheese. Add 2 tsp. vinegar and pinch of chives. Put on top of baked potato.

DIPS, SALADS, DRESSINGS AND SPREADS

Butter Buds Mixture

1 packet of Butter Buds
Safflower Oil (substitute for water in recipe on Butter Buds package)
Stir well and keep refrigerated.
Use in same serving sizes as recommended for margarine.

Sour Cream

Blend 1/3 c. cottage cheese. Add 2 tsp. vinegar and pinch of chives.

"Mayo"

1 c. light mayonnaise
1 c. low-fat cottage cheese
1/4 c. water

Blend cottage cheese and water in blender until smooth. Pour into bowl and mix with the mayonnaise. Put mixture in an empty mayonnaise jar and fool your family!

Slaw

Shredded cabbage (add some grated carrots if desired)
Blend low-fat cottage cheese in blender and add vinegar and Equal to taste for dressing. Mix and refrigerate 1 hour before eating. 1 c. = P.M. (evening) snack or may eat with evening meal.

Whipped Light Cream Cheese

1 c. Philadelphia Light Cream Cheese
1 c. low-fat cottage cheese
1/4 c. water

Blend cottage cheese and water in blender. Pour into bowl with cream cheese and mix well. Store in refrigerator.

Sensational Spinach Dip

Mix onion/cottage cheese dip as per recipe below.
*Add 1/2 pkg. (10 oz.) frozen chopped spinach thawed and squeezed dry.
(*1/2 10 oz. pkg. or double recipe and add whole pkg.)

California Onion Dip

(For raw vegetables)
1 c. blended cottage cheese – low-fat – 1%
2 (rounded) tbsp. onion flakes - dehydrated
1 (rounded) tsp. beef bouillon crystals

Mix and let stand 15-20 minutes before using. Use 1/3 c. per serving.

Tossed Salads

Use any raw veggies and avoid "toppings" (croutons, bacon bits, etc.). Use "carry-with-you" dressing or #3 salad dressing below.

Salad Dressings

Sprinkle salad with vinegar or lemon juice and 2 packets Equal sweetener plus 1 Sweet 'N Low and a pinch of salt. This is best, but for a variety try the following occasionally.

1. Mix 1 1/2 tbsp. Kraft Creamy Italian Low Calorie dressing with 2 tbsp. vinegar, 1 tbsp. water, 1 tbsp. blended cottage cheese and 2-3 packets Equal plus a dash of salt. Use this amount for one salad.

2. Blue Cheese – 1/3 c. cottage cheese – blend in blender. Add 1 1/2 tbsp. (rounded) crumbled blue cheese and dash of salt. Use on one salad.

3. When eating out:

   1 tbsp. any salad dressing – drizzle over salad
   sprinkle vinegar generously over all
   small amount of salt
   2 Equal (as desired) over all (carry this with you)

Ranch Salad Dressing or Dip

1 1/4 c. non-fat milk
1/2 c. "Mayo" (see recipe)

1/4 c. low-fat cottage cheese
1 pkg. reduced calorie Ranch salad
     dressing mix

Blend all ingredients in blender for 60 seconds. Refrigerate 30 minutes before serving to allow dressing to thicken. Stir before serving. Dressing will stay fresh 2-3 weeks. May use up to 1/3 c. per serving.

DESSERTS AND SNACKS

Carrot Cake Squares

1 c. flour	1 packet Butter Buds
1 1/4 tsp. baking powder	1/2 c. water
1/2 tsp. baking soda	2 egg whites, beaten
1/4 tsp. cinnamon	1 c. grated carrots
1/8 tsp. nutmeg	1/3 c. raisins
1/8 tsp. salt	3 Sweet 'n Low
2 tbsp. fructose	5 Equal

Spray square cake pan (8-10 inch) with non-stick spray. Set oven at 350 degrees. Combine all_dry ingredients. Mix water, egg whites, carrots and raisins. Add to dry ingredients and mix thoroughly. Pour into pan and bake at 350 degrees for 30 minutes. Remove from oven and cool 15-20 minutes. Cut into 2 inch squares. Eat as is or split square and put 1-2 tbsp. Whipped Light Cream Cheese (see recipe) on each half. One 2 inch square (with or without cream cheese) makes one evening snack or one lunch dessert.

Cheese Cake

Mix 1 1/4 crushed Sunflakes with 2 tbsp. Butter Buds powder and 3 Equal. Moisten mixture with 1 tbsp. water and 1 tbsp. Safflower oil. Press into bottom of 6 inch pie pan for crust.

Sprinkle 1/2 package Knox plain gelatin on 1/2 c. cool water. Let stand 3 minutes. Heat until gelatin dissolves. Set aside.

Blend in blender:
1 8 oz. package plus 1/4 c. Philadelphia Light Cream Cheese
gelatin and water mixture
1/2 c. low-fat cottage cheese
1 tsp. pure vanilla extract
1 egg
2 tbsp. fructose

Pour into pan. Over low heat bring to very <u>slow</u> simmer <u>stirring constantly</u>. Simmer <u>slowly</u> 2 minutes. Cool and add 6 packets of Equal. Pour into crust and chill until firm. 1/8 of pie = 1 serving.

Chocolate Mousse

1/4 c. cold water
3/4 c. hot water
2 packets chocolate Alba 77
   High Calcium Shake

1/4 tsp. pure vanilla
1 Equal and 1 Sweet 'n Low
1 heaping tbsp. 100% Egg Protein Powder
1/2 package Knox plain gelatin

Soften gelatin in cold water. Add to hot water and heat until thoroughly dissolved. Pour gelatin mixture and rest of ingredients into blender. Blend well and place in refrigerator until firm. 1/3 of recipe = 1 P.M. snack, dinner or lunch dessert.

"E.Z." Sweet Snack

Toasted English Muffin, toasted bagel, or whole grain bread – spread with 1 tsp. diet margarine, sprinkle with Equal – tastes like jelly! If you are eating out, have this when others are having dessert.

Fudge

1 package Alba High Calcium Shake – chocolate
1 tsp. 100% Egg Protein Powder
3 tbsp. peanut butter
1/4 tsp. pure vanilla extract
1 package Nestle's Quick - sugar free
1/3 c. water
1 tbsp. Butter Buds powder
2 tbsp. fat-free dry milk powder
1 tsp. fructose

Mix all ingredients except peanut butter. Heat over lowest heat until smooth, stirring constantly. Remove from heat and stir in peanut butter until smooth. Pour onto flat saucer lined with clear plastic wrap and freeze. When frozen, remove from freezer, let stand 5 minutes and slice into squares – approximately 30. 1 serving = 3 pieces. Store in freezer.

Note: Oatmeal in this recipe tastes good! Add 1 c. oatmeal (long cooking) after peanut butter, drop by teaspoonfuls onto saucer and freeze. Store in freezer.

Fudgesicles

1 c. water
2 packets Alba 77 High Calcium Shake - chocolate
1/4 tsp. pure vanilla
1 packet Equal and 1 Sweet 'n Low
1 heaping tbsp. 100% Egg Protein Powder

Blend in blender and pour into popsicle freezer containers. 2 for evening snack.

Jello or Knox Blocks

2 c. boiling water
1 package plain gelatin

Mix until gelatin is dissolved and add 1 package cherry Nutra Sweet Kool Aid Powder.

Top with blended cottage cheese, mixed with vanilla and Equal or plain cottage cheese (1/4 c.)

Use 2 packages plain gelatin for "Knox Blocks."

Strawberry, Blueberry or Peach Jelly

2 c. strawberries, blueberries, or peaches and juice of 1/2 lemon – place in pan and simmer. Dissolve 1 packet Knox plain gelatin in 1/4 c. cool water. Add to fruit and heat to dissolve gelatin. Cool and add 8 packets Equal sweetener and 4 Sweet 'n Low, sprinkle salt and 2 tbsp. fructose. Cool. Store in refrigerator. Tastes so good, you'll have to make extra for your family! Eat as desired on pancakes, toast, etc., or use as "topping" for cottage cheese instead of "sugary" apple butter!

Peach Fluff Pie

1 can (16 oz.) sugar-free peach halves or slices
1 c. crushed Sunflakes mixed with 2 tbsp. water
2 tbsp. fructose
10 Equal
1 envelope unflavored gelatin
2 tbsp. lemon juice
1/8 tsp. almond extract
1 c. fat-free yogurt
3 egg whites

Drain peaches – save liquid. Blend peaches in blender. In saucepan, place peach liquid, sprinkle with gelatin. Let stand 5 minutes. Heat peach liquid/gelatin mixture over medium heat until gelatin dissolves, stirring occasionally. Blend in blender: peaches, fructose, 6 Equal, lemon juice and almond extract. Chill until mixture is slightly thickened, about 25 minutes. Blend in yogurt; chill. Beat egg whites with electric mixer at high speed. Sprinkle in 2 packets Equal and continue beating until stiff peaks form. Fold into peach mixture; chill until mixture mounds when dropped from spoon, about 1 hour. Press crushed Sunflakes, 2 Equal and water mixture into bottom of pie pan for crust and pour peach filling onto the crust. Chill 4 hours and serve.
1/8 pie = P.M. snack. 1/6 pie = daytime or P.M. snack or lunch dessert.

Strawberry "Short Cake" Pie

21/2 c. sliced unsweetened strawberries
1 tbsp. safflower oil
2 c. Sunflakes crushed
1 tbsp. Butter Buds Powder
2 tbsp. fructose
9 Equal
1 envelope unflavored gelatin
2 tbsp. lemon juice
2 c. low-fat cottage cheese
1/4 tsp. pure vanilla extract

Sprinkle gelatin over 1/4 c. cool water in saucepan. Let stand 5 minutes. Mash with fork, 1/2 c. of the strawberries. Add 1 tbsp. fructose and set aside. Add 1 tbsp. fructose and 6 Equal to remainder of the berries. Mix and set aside. Heat gelatin/water mixture until gelatin dissolves. Remove from heat and add mashed berries and mix well. Add 2 Equal, remainder of sliced berries and lemon juice. Mix well. Chill until mixture is thickened but will still pour. (1 hour). Mix crushed Sunflakes with Butter Buds, 3 Equal and 1 tbsp. water and 1 tbsp. safflower oil, and press into bottom of pie pan. Pour strawberries into crust and chill 4 hours. Blend in blender: 2 c. cottage cheese, 2 tsp. vanilla extract and 4 packets Equal. Spread on top of pie, chill and serve.
1/8 pie = P.M. snack or lunch dessert. 1/5 of pie = afternoon snack.

Quick Strawberry Short Cake

3-4 Equal
2 pancakes (see recipe in "Breakfast Foods")
1/4 c. strawberries, sliced
1/3 c. low-fat cottage cheese

Mix 3-4 Equal with berries and stir. Let stand 10 minutes. Put pancakes on saucer, add berries and top with cottage cheese. Use for lunch dessert. Use one pancake for P.M. snack. Use 4 pancakes for afternoon snack.

Rice Pudding

1 c. rice
2 c. water
1/2 tsp. salt

Boil until tender, approximately 15-20 minutes and rinse in cold water. Drain. Return to pot and add:

2 c. non-fat milk	3 Sweet 'n Low
1 1/2 c. water	1/3 c. raisins
2 tbsp. Butter Buds Powder	2 tbsp. fructose

Simmer 15-20 minutes stirring occasionally. Cool 5 minutes and add 4-6 Equal and stir. Cool in serving dish, sprinkle with cinnamon and refrigerate. 1/2 c. = afternoon snack.

Topping for Cottage Cheese or Yogurt
(Eat as Desired)

3 c. water
1 package plain gelatin
2 packages Nutra Sweet Kool-Aid, any flavor desired
2 tsp. fructose

Soften gelatin in 1 c. water. Add to 2 c. boiling water. Simmer and stir until gelatin is dissolved, 3-5 minutes. Add fructose, cool and add Kool-Aid powder (2 packages). Refrigerate until "set." *Use as desired for "topping" on low-fat cottage cheese or yogurt.

*Also – see recipe for jelly and use as topping.

Yogurt/Grape Nuts Snack
(A.M. or P.M. Snack)

1/2 c. yogurt – sweeten with Equal

Add 1 <u>heaping</u> tsp. Grape Nuts cereal. Let stand 2-3 minutes.

"Cream" of Tomato Soup

3/4 c. (or small 6 oz. can) tomato juice
3 tbsp. water
1 tsp. powdered non-dairy coffee creamer <u>or</u> non-fat milk powder
1 Equal
sprinkle of salt (optional)

Heat tomato juice and water until hot. Pour into mug and add creamer (or milk powder), Equal and salt. Have with 1/2 slice low-fat cheese on 1 Wasa bread or 2 melba for evening snack.

"Melba" Toast

4 slices diet whole wheat bread toasted <u>lightly</u>. Cut down middle of each slice to make 8 thin slices. Toast lightly again. Cool and cut each thin slice in half to make 16 pieces. Store in plastic food bag.

Morning Apple/Cheese Snack

1 slice low-fat cheese
1 apple (small) sliced

Cut cheese slice into thirds. Cut again across the thirds to six equal pieces. Cut apple into 6 slices. Place 1 piece of cheese on each.

Sweet Cucumbers

sliced fresh cucumbers
1 c. vinegar
6-8 Equal

1/2 c. water
1 tbsp. dehydrated onion flakes

Mix vinegar, water, Equal and dehydrated onion flakes. Pour over sliced cucumbers in pint jar. Cover and refrigerate overnight. Will keep 1 month or more. Tastes like sweet pickles. Eat as desired, anytime.

Waldorf Salad

1/2 small apple, chopped
1/3 c. low-fat cottage cheese
1/2 tbsp. raisins
1 Equal

Mix all ingredients. Makes 1 serving.

Whipped Light Cream Cheese

Blend in blender – 1 c. low-fat cottage cheese and 3 tbsp. water. Remove from blender and mix in large bowl with 1 c. light cream cheese. Let stand in refrigerator several hours before eating.

Note – may <u>double</u> light cream cheese serving sizes when using this recipe.

Yogurt & Strawberries or Peaches

1/4 c. strawberries or peaches – fresh or unsweetened frozen
1 c. low-fat yogurt
4 Equal and 2 Sweet 'n Low (adjust to sweetness desired)

12

RESISTANCE TO FIRM, TONE AND RESHAPE

Your activity – walking and using the mini tramp at your exercise heart rate is called "aerobic" exercise. Nothing can reduce body fat or improve the cardio-vascular system as efficiently as aerobic exercise. However, resistance exercise, using weights to provide resistance for body muscles, is the only way to firm, tone and reshape the body. When muscles are not exercised adequately using resistance, they will atrophy (shrink) contributing to the look we all know too well as "flab."

I have included resistance exercise at this point, not because you should begin after you have lost weight and are ready for maintenance, but simply because it is best not to take on too much at one time. Allow yourself four to five weeks to adjust to your eating and activity plan and then add a resistance exercise program if you want the very best results you can get. While it is not an absolute necessity, adding resistance exercise is highly recommended. It not only assists with fat loss, but it will be a definite asset in helping maintain your weight loss.

The Need For Resistance Exercise

Muscle tone is the crowning glory of an attractive body. Adding resistance exercise will keep the body healthy and young looking as it shapes, contours and improves muscle tone and firmness.

When young, you have firm, healthy muscles, but muscles atrophy faster and faster as you get beyond your 20's. Developing and keeping muscles firm and healthy through resistance exercise will make you look younger and shapelier at any age. Shaping the entire body and recontouring problem areas, these exercises help increase flexibility, rehabilitate injured or weak body parts, and will also aid osteoporosis and arthritis victims. It has become apparent that most people using a weight program feel better, sleep better, have more sexual drive and look better.

Women and Weights

Occasionally, a woman will shun weight training for fear of building bulky muscles, a fear that is totally unfounded. A woman does not have enough male sex hormones to grow huge muscles no matter how hard she tries. In fact, it is not unusual for women in their 40's and 50's to have younger and shapelier bodies as a result of their resistance exercise training. Unlike men, women usually look smaller, as fat is reduced and "saddlebags" and "cellulite" disappear. "Proof of the pudding" is that today's top fashion models, both men and women, are very much aware of the benefits and use resistance exercise to insure their modeling careers by keeping their bodies firm, healthy and attractive.

If for no other reason, it is important that women use resistance exercise to ward off osteoporosis. Bone loss in women begins in the 30's and between 30 and 50 there is a loss of about one percent of their bone mass per year. This loss will accelerate when they pass through menopause. Resistance exercise will increase bone density which will prevent or halt the progress of osteoporosis.

So that you do not misunderstand, *adding* not *substituting* resistance exercise is the recommendation. Let me give you a brief summary of the many advantages of adding resistance exercise to your activity program.

Advantages of Resistance Exercise

a. One pound of fat takes up five times the space of one pound of lean muscle. As body fat is lost and lean muscle increases, inches are lost and the body becomes firmed and toned.

b. There will be a total reshaping of the body or parts of the body.

c. Muscle tissue burns more calories than fat tissue, therefore, increasing muscle tissue as fat is decreased can mean a smaller, firmer body that not only burns more calories at rest, but also burns more calories for each and every activity.

d. Resistance exercise increases bone density – a big plus for bone strength for all, especially for women who are prone to osteoporosis.

e. There are special benefits for women. The female hormonal system does not support large increases in muscle size. Losing body fat while using resistance exercise to firm and tone helps decrease overall body size, firm and uplift the bust, buttocks, and underarm "flab," while improving posture and strength.

f. There are special benefits for men. Resistance exercise will help reshape the male body to produce the broad shouldered, narrow wasted "v" shape most men desire. The male hormonal system supports production of more muscle mass and upper body strength than that of the female. Some men may want to produce more muscle than others, and their resistance exercise program should be based on personal preferences.

One word of caution. Resistance exercise gives excellent results when performed correctly. It can also cause serious injury if performed incorrectly. Be sure to seek out professional guidance and instruction at a highly qualified fitness center when beginning a resistance exercise program. Make sure the fitness center you choose offers a short-term membership contract such as three or six months. This will allow you a trial period to experience the kind of service you will be getting before obligating yourself for a long period of time.

Questions
Resistance to Firm, Tone and Reshape

I'm over 50 years of age and have never lifted weights before. Isn't it too late for me to try resistance exercise?

No. It is never too late! Research has shown that resistance exercise can help build lean body tissue and strengthen bones, no matter what your age. Of course, a 60 or 70 year old will not see results as quickly as a 30 year old, nevertheless, firming, reshaping and strength gains do occur. The most important thing to remember is to start slowly and gradually work up to the intensity of each exercise. Better yet, investigate a good fitness center – one that offers individual programs with qualified instructors.

Won't women become too muscular and end up looking like men if they use weights?

What many people fail to realize is that women do not have the amount of male hormones required to develop the muscles men have. Another point to remember, there are specific lifting exercises for specific goals. Weight training can be designed for toning and firming without developing big muscles.

It is not hard to find some good books on resistance exercises for women, or join a fitness center. A word of caution on fitness centers – some are excellent, some are not. Make sure the following is available before you join:

1. A short-term membership of 3 or 6 months that will allow you time to try out the facility before making long-term financial commitments.
2. A monitoring plan to monitor your progress and change your exercise program on a regular basis throughout your entire membership.
3. An exercise program designed for you based on your needs, which must include three components: 1) aerobic exercise, 2) resistance exercise and 3) nutrition guidelines. A nutritionist on staff is an excellent bonus!

I play tennis and I don't want to become "muscle bound" from lifting weights. Won't lifting weights ruin my tennis game?

Twenty years or more ago people who lifted weights were considered a little "strange." Many coaches wouldn't let their athletes lift because they would become "muscle bound." Today, most top athletes and teams have a weight training program. Research has shown that fewer injuries occur and performance improves with a proper strength training program. If you lift correctly, your tennis game will improve and you'll end up being stronger.

Isn't a good aerobics program and a good nutrition program enough for losing weight and looking fit?

Since body fat takes up *five* times as much space as lean body tissue, losing 40 or 60 pounds, for example, is going to leave a lot of sagging skin and muscles. It is important to firm your body and the only way to firm and reshape problem areas is through resistance exercise. While aerobic exercise is excellent for reducing body fat, for a total body shape up, you must also include resistance exercise.

Is it true that in lifting weights, the breasts can become larger?

This is only partly true. Since breasts contain a large percent of fat, the loss of fat may reduce the breast area. However, lifting weights can build up the muscles under the breasts (pectorals) which will uplift the breast area and make the breasts firmer, and *appear* larger if they were small to begin with. However, large breasts have a larger amount of fat and the above process will not compensate for a large amount of fat loss.

I have a bad back. Can I lift weights?

This is an area that has to be fully investigated. There are cases where certain back problems prevent the use of resistance exercises. However, in the majority of cases, a properly designed resistance program can help back problems. Just remember, if your back muscles are weak, the spine will not have adequate support to help keep it healthy and strong.

Is it necessary to continue to lift weights after the toning and shape up is successful?

It is a fact that the human body is designed to be active. If muscles aren't exercised, they become "slack" and begin to atrophy. Humans must have some form of activity in order to look and be healthy. Resistance exercise is an activity that can be done throughout your entire lifetime. Using weights is an excellent activity which produces positive results. Weight training can also be easily combined with other activities. Accept the fact that exercise must be done for the rest of your life or your body will not stay in peak condition!

Joining a fitness club is too expensive. Suppose I can't afford to join a center or gym?

Joining a fitness club is really not expensive if you shop for a club that gives you service and has individualized programs. If you can't find the money to join, go to the book store and get a good basic book on resistance exercise. It isn't necessary to purchase a lot of expensive equipment either, just a basic weight set or dumbbell set. If you can't afford these, use some empty bleach bottles or detergent bottles and fill them with water and use as resistance weights. For light weights use less water, for heavier weights, use more water.

13

SPECIAL HELPS

In this chapter you will find information that will be of special interest to assist in reaching your goal. Most of this information is geared to help you focus on the important aspects of weight control, while some will be useful in evaluating your progress. People who have gone through the "Fat To Fit Without Dieting" program felt the "Special Helps" information in this chapter to be some of the most useful in their continuing progress.

Included is "Helpful Hints" which illustrates two examples of adjustments for meals and snacks to suit different schedules, and is also a quick reminder of some important aspects of your program.

"Things You Need to Know to Change Your Lifestyle to Slim Forever" lists dietary guidelines of the eating plan and questions you will want to be able to answer plus brief "Activity Guidelines."

"Guidelines—Losing and Maintaining" is a condensed view with brief listings of important guidelines while losing and while maintaining, followed by brief check points if you begin to gain.

The "Daily Evaluation" is a game type approach to score your daily progress. It will assist in checking your intake of dietary fat, simple and complex carbohydrates and water as well as your eating habits and activity plan. Use this handy little scoring sheet daily to help keep you "on track"!

"Good For You Sweets" is a list of sweets for the occasional sweet tooth, or for those of you who want healthy refreshments for guests when entertaining.

"Did You Know" presents some interesting information in question form about obesity, cellulite, etc.

Ending the chapter is "Twenty Questions," a list of the most frequently asked questions with answers following, to help with everyday situations such as dining at a friend's, getting hungry in the evening, losing weight faster, etc.

It is recommended that you make a copy of those selections you find most helpful and carry them with you or post in a conspicuous place for convenient reference.

HELPFUL HINTS

Helpful Hints

1. Breakfast and Lunch – Largest Meals of Day
    Think in terms of planning your dinner when planning lunch. What you normally have for dinner will most likely make an excellent lunch.

2. Dinner (Supper) – Smallest Meal of Day
    Think in terms of planning your lunch when planning your dinner. If your family rebels and insists on a large "meat and potatoes" evening meal, don't fight them! You may eat with them, but modify. Put a small serving of each food on a small bread dish for yourself. Have an acidophilus shake or large tossed salad on the side. Or have a *large* serving of the veggies you've cooked and a very *small* portion of the meat, and always have an appetizer.

3. Snacks Are a Must!
    If you have a busy schedule, keep snacks simple, convenient AND always on hand – a bagel, bread with 2 teaspoons peanut butter or 1 slice low-fat cheese, etc.

4. Plan Meals and Snacks to Fit Conveniently in Schedule
    Eating must occur every 21/2-3 hours. Eat on your way to or from work. Keep convenient non-perishable snacks in your car if you travel a lot. If you like oatmeal, fix enough for breakfast and afternoon snack – take it in a small thermos for afternoon snack. The following are examples of changes made to fit meals and snacks into schedules conveniently:

Darlene M.'s schedule modified to suit her best!
Up @ 5:30 A.M. – have WW bread and 4 amino acid tablets
Begin fast walk @ 5:45 A.M.
Back home @ 6:50 A.M. – shower and dress
Leave for work @ 7:40 A.M. – take breakfast along
Arrive @ work @ 8:40 A.M. – eat breakfast - nice break before work!
11:30 A.M. – eat lunch
2:00 P.M. – snack (light)
4:30 P.M. – snack (complex carbohydrate)
6:30 P.M. – eat dinner (light)
9:30 P.M. – bed

John R.'s schedule is unpredictable – modified to suit him best!
1. Plan menu 1 week in advance
2. Plan <u>times</u> of snacks and meals 1 day in advance based upon appointments for the day.
3. Carry non-perishable snacks in car when on the road.
4. Eat oatmeal and amino acid tablets at home and take
    English muffin along to eat on the way for breakfast or for snack.

THINGS YOU NEED

TO KNOW TO CHANGE

YOUR LIFESTYLE

TO SLIM

FOREVER

Things You Need To Know
To Change Your Lifestyle
To Slim Forever

Check your "Fat To Fit" knowledge with the following. Look up anything you feel unsure about.

Low Fat	1.	What foods are high in fat; low in fat?
	2.	How to lower fat intake.
	3.	Substitutions for high fat foods.
High Fiber	1.	What foods are high in fiber?
	2.	Complex vs. simple carbohydrates.
	3.	High fiber snacks.
High Complex Carbohydrates	1.	What are complex carbohydrate foods?
	2.	Complex vs. simple carbohydrates.
	3.	Complex carbohydrate snacks.
Moderate Protein	1.	What are protein foods?
	2.	How often to eat.
	3.	How to get needed Amino Acids, without increasing protein/fat intake.
Water	1.	How to increase intake of water.
	2.	Importance of.
	3.	How much needed?
Three Meals, Three Snacks Daily	1.	Importance of snacks.
	2.	What kinds of snacks?
	3.	When to snack.
	4.	Breakfast is a <u>must</u> – why?
	5.	Evening meal – lightest of day – why?
	6.	Never stuffed, never hungry.

Activity Planning Guidelines

Fast Walk or Mini Trampoline	1.	Importance of.
	2.	How Activity Plan works with Eating Plan to correct overweight.
	3.	How to begin.
	4.	How to compute and monitor Exercise Heart Rate.
	5.	Warm-up and cool down.
	6.	Stretching – importance of how to.
	7.	How and when to increase intensity and duration of activity.

IMPORTANT POINTS –

LOSING & MAINTAINING

Important Points – Losing & Maintaining

While Losing Body Fat:

1. Fruit (raw is best) – limit to 6 small pieces/week.
2. Three meals and three snacks/day is best.
   Never omit afternoon snack.
3. Limit – one P/F meal and one P/F snack daily.
4. Omit desserts for a minimum of 4-6 weeks.
5. Writing "Eating Plan" one week in advance is best.
6. Eat only foods you enjoy.
7. Have a *minimum* of *one* raw vegetable snack daily.
8. Evening meal – smaller "lunch type" meal;
   lunch – largest meal of day.
9. Use "Quick Weight Loss" to remedy overindulgences.
10. Never hungry, never stuffed!
11. Activity goal – 1 hour daily.

To Maintain:

1. Best to continue 3 meals and 2-3 snacks – *never* omit afternoon snack.
2. Evening meal – smallest of day; lunch largest.
3. "Binge" day once weekly or as tolerated.
4. P/F meals and snacks – increase occasionally to 2/day if tolerated.
5. *Plan* meals and snacks one day in advance.
6. Increase fruit gradually as tolerated.
7. Eat only foods you enjoy!
8. Never hungry, never stuffed!
9. Use "Quick Weight Loss" to remedy overindulgences.
10. Activity – minimum 50-60 minutes, 3-4 times weekly.
    Adjust if necessary.

If You Begin To Gain – Check Points:

1. Fruit intake
2. Activity and EHR
3. Evening meals
4. P/F meals and snacks
5. Fiber intake
6. Snacks (especially afternoon)

DAILY EVALUATION

Daily Evaluation

The Daily Evaluation will help simplify your Fat To Fit program, allowing you to focus on the six basic areas, and areas where you may need help.

Fat To Fit – Getting & Staying Fit

1. Dietary Fat   Points
   a. Had nothing fried or prepared
      with butter, oil or fat.   5
   b. Had only low-fat dairy products:
      low-fat cheese slices, low-fat cottage
      cheese, fat-free yogurt, butter buds,
      2 tbsp. or less of Light cream cheese,
      etc.   5
   c. Had margarine and/or salad
      dressings according to amounts
      permitted on Eating Plan.   5

   Possible Score: 15   Total Score _____

2. Simple Carbohydrates
   a. Had no sugar products, deserts etc.   10
   b. Had no foods that had added sugar.   3
   c. Had less than one average serving
      of food with added sugar.   2

   Possible Score: 15   Total Score _____

3. Complex Carbohydrates & Fiber
   a. Breads I had were all whole grain.   3
   b. Had whole grain snacks and/or
      permitted fruit and vegetable snacks.   4
   c. Had minimum of 1 raw vegetable or
      1 raw fruit snack.   4
   d. Had minimum of 4 servings vegetables.   4

   Possible Score: 15   Total Score _____

4. Water
   a. Had 6 or more cups.   5
   b. Had 4 cups.   3
   c. Had 3 cups.   2

   Possible Score: 5   Total Score _____

5. Eating Thin
   a. Was not stuffed; was not hungry
      after meals.   5
   b. Had three meals and the smallest
      was in the evening.   5
   c. Afternoon snack included.   5
   d. Evening snack was smallest of the day.   5

   Possible Score: 20   Total Score _____

6. Activity Plan**
   a. 35-40 minutes   20
   b. 41-50 minutes   30
   c. 51-60 minutes   40
   d. Over 60 minutes   45

   Possible Score: 45   Total Score _____

** At Exercise Heart Rate (see p. 67) – do not include warm up
in total time listed above.

Possible Total Score: 115   Total Score – ALL _____

A score of 115 every day is not necessary. If you consistently score *above* 95 you will probably still lose weight. If you "slip" and score below 95 try to get a higher score the next day or two to compensate. Remember, you are human and you will have occasional "slips" which are not the problem as much as *what you do afterwards*! If you get back to your Eating Plan the next day, and add an *extra* session of activity for a day or two, you will remedy the "slip." Remember that these are bound to occur and even the most successful weight loss people have had "slips" on occasion. Be prepared to "undo" them with extra Activity time and extra diligence with your Eating Plan for three or four days afterward, or follow the "Quick Weight Loss Plan" for a short period of time.

GOOD FOR YOU

SWEETS

Good For You Sweets
(For Evening Snacking)

Most people find that their taste for sweets is greatly reduced after two or three weeks on the Eating Plan. However, when there are occasions that the taste buts (not appetite) want a little something sweet, here are some evening snacks that will not interfere with weight loss. As a bonus, these sweets are actually good for you!

Be sure to plan and *prepare ahead of time*! One of the greatest appeals of cakes, cookies, etc., is their convenience. It is much easier to reach into a box of cookies than to take the time to prepare something, especially in the evening.

Don't overlook these delicious dishes when planning refreshments for your guests if you entertain. And do invite your family to enjoy these snacks with you. It will be much healthier for them and you may not be asked to keep other tempting foods on hand.

Keep sweet snacks occasional. If you are the kind of person who, once started on sweet tasting food, has difficulty stopping with just one serving, then it may be better to wait several weeks or months before having them.

Good "Sweets" For Occasional Evening Snacks, Lunch Desserts or Entertaining

(Post on Refrigerator Door)

1. *Peach Fluff Pie 1/6 pie
2. 1 thin slice whole wheat bread w/ 2 tsp. peanut butter and *jelly
3. *Fudge – 2 pieces
4. *Fudgesicles - 2
5. 1/3 c. low-fat cottage cheese w/ *jelly
6. *Cinnamon toast (2 thin)
7. *Acidophilus "Snack" Shake
8. 3 *melba w/ *jelly
9. 1/3 c. low-fat cottage cheese w/ 1/4 c. sugar-free   peaches. Sweeten w/ Equal

10. *Strawberry Short Cake Pie 1/6 pie
11. *jello w/ low-fat cottage cheese topping
12. 1 c. *slaw
13. *sweet cucumber pickles
14. *pancakes (2) w/ *jelly
15. *Carrot Cake Squares (one 2 inch square)
16. 1/3 c. Sunflakes w/ 1/3 c. non-fat milk
17. 1/2 c. *non-fat yogurt w/ sugar-free strawberries
18. 1/2 c. non-fat yogurt w/ 1 tbsp. Grapenuts or Nutri Grain Nuggets and 2-3 Equal
19. 2 *pancakes w/ 1/4 c. low-fat cottage cheese, topped w/ sugar-free strawberries. Sweeten w/ Equal
20. 1/2 c. strawberries w/ 1/3 c. low-fat cottage cheese(sweeten berries w/ Equal)
21. *Cheese Cake 1/8 pie (limit 2x week)

*   See Recipe

DID YOU KNOW?

FAT FACTS – CAN YOU

SEPARATE FACT FROM

FICTION?

Did You Know?
Fat Facts – Can You Separate Fact From Fiction?

Obesity is caused by eating too much.

This statement is false! There are many causes, all of which have one common denominator – a slow metabolism! The fact is that we now know that obesity is not caused simply by overeating.

Getting rid of cellulite takes special techniques.

Not so! Cellulite is fat that causes dimpling of the skin as it pushes up between connective tissue under the skin. It is not a special "toxic waste" of the body but good (or bad) old body fat. The same eating plan and activity plan that gets rid of body fat will also get rid of "cellulite."

You do not get rid of fat cells when you lose body fat.

Unfortunately this is true. Fat cells *empty* when fat is lost, but once cells are created they are ours for life, and we can only change the amount of fat that is in them!

Weight gain is especially critical at certain times of our lives.

Yes! During infancy and again during adolescence, fat cells are produced more abundantly than any other period of time. Once the cells are produced they remain for life. For this reason, fat gains especially during adolescence is not to be taken lightly. Once the fat cells are created and body fat is lost these cells will empty but the body has a tendency to attempt to fill the empty cells, making weight control more difficult. Weight control is a smart move for adolescents, and extra "chubby" is out for infants!

The scales are reliable in telling how fat you are.

Absolutely not! Many people of average weight lose body fat (very light in weight) gain lean muscle (heavier in weight) having *no* change in weight but end up smaller around waist and hips with a much firmer, shaplier body. Also, many of our athletes who are very muscular have a very low body fat percentage, but with extra muscle tissue (lean is heavier) weigh more than the ever-popular height/weight tables suggest. Other people look thin, weigh less than they should but have a "flabby" appearance because their body fat percentage in relation to body lean is too high! (Consider the sedentary 75 year old who is thin in appearance but whose body is extremely "flabby" – underweight and overfat!)

Snacking between meals will make you fat.

Not so! Research proves, that eating smaller amounts several times daily produces weight loss whereas one large meal daily increases the tendency to store fat 25 fold. In addition, metabolic increases occur more often and the thermic effect of food "wastes" more calories when eating occurs more often.

Leg exercises are best for fat on legs and stomach exercises are best for fat on the stomach.

No, no, no! Aerobic exercise is necessary to lose fat wherever it is. You can do leg exercises from now until "the cows come home" and you will not get rid of the fat on your legs! Stomach exercises will firm the stomach muscles, but the layer of fat on the top of those muscles will still protrude without aerobic exercise to reduce the fat!

Brown fat is a good fat to have.

Yes! Brown fat is found only in very small quantities and is used primarily for heat production to keep vital body organs warm. Brown fat activity uses calories at a tremendous rate. Dieting not only reduces but in some cases stops brown fat activity!

Certain foods produce more body fat than others.

Yes, indeed! Dietary fat and refined sugar produce more body fat than other foods. Dietary fat does because metabolically it is the easiest food for the body to convert to fat. Remember the statement – "you may as well spread mayonnaise on your hips" – more truth than fiction! And sugar? Sugar precipitates an insulin reaction which not only causes a craving for more, but the insulin itself is a fat promoting hormone causing fat production and fat storage. A double whammy from sugar!

Fat absorption can be decreased with fiber foods.

You bet! Always eat some high fiber foods when you eat foods containing fat – steak with a tossed salad, etc. Even the Pizza Hut now offers a salad bar. Good thinking! Fiber combines with dietary fat and prevents some of its absorption. And I did say *some*, not *all*, so take heed. Adding fiber so you can have *high fiber* fat meals won't work – you'll still get too much fat!

LIVING FIT –
TWENTY QUESTIONS

Living Fit – Twenty Questions

These questions provide excellent reference and review for you. See how many you can answer without looking at the answers. Several of them have more than one answer or different answers than are suggested based on your own situation or on your own food preferences. Use them as often as you need for reference, additional information or review.

1. You're invited to dinner and the hostess has:
    Fried Chicken   Salad
    Green Beans   Chocolate Cake
    Mashed Potatoes Ice Cream

    What to do?

    Answer: Green beans – (non "seed-type" veggie) – large serving.
    Salad – (ask for dressing on the side) – large serving.
    Chicken – (remove skin) – 1-2 pieces.
    Mashed Potatoes – extra small serving.
    Chocolate Cake and Ice Cream – extra small serving or omit.

   If you want to omit the cake and ice cream, use a little psychology. Let me share with you an approach that works very well. You may be able to think of something better, but this has worked in many situations for me.

   If I know there's going to be dessert and I'm not due for a "Binge Day" food, I'll pick a "safe" food and begin, during the meal, to compliment the hostess. "This tossed salad is excellent! I can never make a tossed salad that tastes really good, but this one is outstanding. I don't know what you did, but I have never eaten a salad this good!" When the time comes for dessert, it's time for the "punch line," and it always works. "I never thought I would turn down chocolate cake and ice cream for salad, but yours is the very best I've ever eaten. I can get chocolate cake and ice cream anytime, but I can't get your wonderful salad. Do you mind if I have another salad instead of the ice cream and cake?" Compliments like this are hard to turn down. With this approach you have made your hostess' day and saved yours!

You may also alter the above, ask for just a taste of the cake and ice cream so that you can save room for one more of her delicious salads. You may also plan ahead and have this dinner for your "Binge Day."

Also, do remember to eat something right before leaving home or on the way, anytime you plan to eat out, to take the edge off your appetite making sure it is well under control!

2. You've had a busy day and missed your afternoon snack. It's evening and you're hungry! You've already eaten dinner.

Answer: 1/2 sandwich on diet or thin whole grain bread with tuna or 1/2 low-fat cheese slice and a cup of "cream of tomato" soup (see recipe) is excellent for an emergency like this. Raw veggies may be added if desired. If this doesn't suit your taste, you may want to have a large tossed salad with one of the dressings listed in the recipe section.

3. You're shopping with a friend. It's snack time and you forgot to bring a snack. What to do?

Answer: Food is almost always available when out shopping. You may stop in almost anyplace and order a small "house" salad. Most of our malls now have either baked potato stands (plain with margarine on the side) or popcorn stands (plain, air popped). Grocery stores offer endless choices – bagels, fruit, vegetables, and if nothing else, whole grain bread.

4. You order spaghetti. You've become completely satisfied with 1/2 the order. What to do?

Answer: Doggie Bag! Spaghetti is something I seldom have time to make at home. I order spaghetti for dinner, eat lots of salad and just a very small taste of the spaghetti, doggie bag the remainder and my lunch is ready for the next day! The most delicious lunches I eat come from doggie bags!

5. You have a dinner party – what to serve?

Answer: This should be no problem if you browse through the recipe section. Any lean meat of your choice, non "seed-type" veggies and even dessert (cheese cake is excellent!). If you wish you may also plan your dinner party for your "Binge Day."

6. You have friends over for cards and snacks weekly – what to serve?

Answer: Once again, check your list of "Meals And Snacks – Suggestions." Most people today are more aware of good nutrition and will appreciate veggies and dip as part of the snacks. Also, check "Good For You Sweets" in this chapter.

7. Binge Day – When? What to have? Where are guidelines?

Answer: "Binge Day" should not occur until a minimum of 4-6 weeks after beginning the program, and only then if you feel comfortable in so doing.

In planning what to have, plan one dessert food or one meal for the day that is off limits for you otherwise. You may want a banana split, a chocolate nut sundae, or another favorite dessert food. Some people may prefer lobster tail with butter or another favorite meal, while others may enjoy having potato chips. Your "Binge Day" should include a favorite meal or a favorite food, but is *not* a day in which you "binge" on food all day long! When eating your binge food or meal, eat only until you are comfortable – never stuff yourself!

When to plan? Only after 4-6 weeks on the program and then weekly if desired, but *only* if activity and eating have been "on target" for the entire week.

For guidelines, see "Guidelines For Planning Menus."

8. If you've had a "slip" – what to do?

Answer: The most important thing is not to allow yourself to feel *guilty*! Guilt always compounds the problem – "I've been bad so I may as well be really bad . . ." With this thought you're on your way to "self-destruct." Consider the following example.

An archer's "mistakes" (missing the target) are all part of *learning* to hit the target. Each "miss" helps him/her learn adjustments that are necessary in order to hit the target.

Each "slip" is an opportunity to learn some adjustments that may be necessary for you. Mistakes are excellent learning situations if you will allow them to be. Situations will arise that you are unsure of or that you do not handle as you would have liked. No problem! Walk yourself mentally through the situation the next day and try to discover other alternatives you could have chosen. This is one of my favorite mental exercises. I've designed perhaps as much as a third of the program with help of "slips" I've had in various situations.

In the meantime, you can always undo the "slips" by adding one extra activity session and adhering strictly to the Eating Plan for two or three days. The "Quick Weight Loss" eating and activity has been specifically designed for use after "slips" and results are excellent if followed for several days or a week, to help get you back "on track" and prevent a weight gain. Many people will use this the week before and again after the Christmas and New Years holidays because they choose to have more than one "binge" day during the holiday week and want extra "insurance" to avoid a weight gain.

9. Why is an Activity Plan important?

Answer: The Activity Plan increases fat burning and metabolism with a *bonus* – the fat burning and metabolism increases continue for fifteen to twenty hours *after* the activity is completed! It is important to remember that these increases will occur *only* if the activity is, 1) performed at your exercise heart rate, 2) for a minimum of 30 minutes!

10. Why are pounds lost slower than inches on this plan?

Answer: Pounds are lost slower because you are losing the lightest part of your body – the fat. The good news is that fat takes up a lot of space. One pound of fat takes up *five* times the space of one pound of lean. Want to know how to equate this to pounds lost through a dieting approach? You would have to lose almost *twice* as many pounds dieting, to lose the same number of inches you lose on this plan!

11. Why use the Daily Evaluation?

Answer: The *Daily Evaluation* helps you to focus on the important aspects of the program and will also help you identify your weaknesses as well as your strengths.

Most people write their scores on a separate piece of paper so they can use the Daily Evaluation over again each day.

12. You feel like having a steak. When is best and what with it?

Answer: Steak that is broiled with fat removed is good to have for lunch or Sunday dinner. Have a baked potato with 1 tbsp. sour cream (more if using sour cream recipe) and a tossed salad (for fiber to help prevent some of the fat absorption).

13. What 2 kinds of foods are the best sources of Complex Carbohydrates?

Answer: Complex Carbohydrates – 1) vegetables, and 2) anything made from grains (breads, cereals, popcorn, etc.).

14. Complex Carbohydrate foods are usually high _____ foods also.

Answer: Fiber!

15. Why eat high fiber foods?

Answer: High fiber foods will help assist weight loss in basically three ways:
1. Not calorie dense, they fill you up, not out! These foods take up a lot of space in your stomach and give you a full feeling on far fewer calories.
2. Increase food transit time. Food passes through your body and is eliminated quicker, allowing less time for fat and calorie absorption.
3. Fiber is insoluble and will combine with the fat in your meal, preventing some of its absorption. This is an excellent reason for always including some fiber with meals that have fat!

16. Why is it a good idea to have a few carrots or celery strips or other raw veggies with lunch and dinner?

    Answer: Fiber! These raw veggies will prevent the absorption of some of the fat of your lunch and dinner meals!

17. Are there any foods you have to totally omit on this plan?

    Answer: No! Modify, do not eliminate foods you like. If you love potato chips or ice cream, plan to have some on your "Binge Day!"

18. What will increase metabolism and the body's rate of fat burning? For how long?

    Answer: The activity, done a minimum of 30 minutes at your EHR increases metabolism and fat burning for 15-20 hours (thirty lashes with a wet noodle if you missed this one!).

19. What happens if your metabolism is slower than normal?

    Answer: Calories are burned slower leaving more for fat storage and less for energy. Weight increases and energy decreases, each enhancing the other in compounding weight control problems. Dieting (an artificial food shortage) will intensify energy decreases as well as fat production as the metabolism slows even more, conserving as much as possible to prevent starvation.

20. What is the only way to speed up weight loss if you wish to lose more than 1-2 pounds/week.

    Answer: Increasing activity time or the "Quick Weight Loss" program. *Never* cut calories alone, or you will slow the metabolism as discussed in question #19.

    The best approach is to keep an eye on the *inches* you're losing. Choose a particular size of clothing you would like to comfortably fit into and make that your goal rather than a predetermined weight. The scales weigh whatever is put on them. If you drink two large glasses of water, you will weigh more, but that doesn't mean you've gained weight! Don't get into the "trap" of basing your success totally on the scales. Keep your eye on your goal — increasing metabolism through a change in lifestyle habits. Making comfortable changes gradually to those you enjoy and are happy with should be your goal, and the pounds that come off, as a result, will be off *permanently*. Five months will be here when five months have passed no matter what you do. You will either be thinner than you are now or not. Don't hurry!

My own philosophy — accomplishing anything in a hurry requires a sacrifice in quality and permanence!

14

MAINTENANCE

Rest assured that maintenance is surprisingly easy and if you are a previous dieter, you will find it very different than expected. A dieting maintenance program requires subsisting the rest of your life on very restrictive calorie intakes, or . . . gain back the weight! But, now you have the information and the knowledge to compensate when necessary and adjust to suit you and your lifestyle best.

Before listing maintenance guidelines it is important to look at the variations in approaches to maintenance by those who have lost weight and kept it off. While alterations in lifestyle habits are necessary, they must be workable for you – convenient and tailored to your schedule and needs. Therefore, each maintenance program needs to be individualized and as such will vary based on each individual's needs and preferences. Let's look at some examples.

Examples Of Maintenance Program

The first is a woman in her late forties who maintains her weight at 128 pounds, from a former 175 pounds. She has three meals plus an afternoon snack and includes some kind of dessert three days a week. She compensates by doing her mini trampoline activity 60 minutes five times weekly plus an extra 25 minute walk at lunch. She feels the dessert is worth the extra activity. However, *when she misses two or more of her activity times she omits the desserts or she will gain weight.* The eating plan plus the extra activity gives her the metabolic increase she needs to avoid weight gain even with dessert three times a week.

The second is a man who has a severe weight problem, and needed to lose 160 pounds. He had dieted and gone on extended "fasts" so many times that his metabolic rate was extremely low when he entered the program. He could not tolerate a "binge" food or meal for two months without a weight gain, although by that time, he was walking daily 1 hour in the morning plus a 30 minute evening walk and later added a 1-1/2 hour weight training program three times a week! He didn't complain because for the first time in his life, he was losing weight without hunger and eating more food, even without the "binge," than he ever had on any of his starvation diets. By the third month he had added a "binge" meal without a weight gain and continued to lose to his desired weight. He continues his one hour walk, each day, adds another half hour walk two or three times a week plus his 1-1/2 hour weight training program three times a week. Even with all the extra activity, this man has no desire to return to old habits which had caused hypertension, extreme fatigue (afternoon naps had been absolutely necessary just to function all day) and embarrassment at his tremendous body size which would not fit into regular sized chairs. His blood pressure medication has been discontinued, triglycerides and cholesterol both are back to normal and he enjoys an energy level he has never known before.

To the other extreme, there have been a few people who follow the basic eating plan, have three meals and afternoon snacks, eat satisfying amounts of the foods they like, and find that they must restrict their aerobic activity to three or four 40 minute sessions to prevent losing too much weight! This happens more often to men in their 30's or younger, who have less weight at the start to lose and who have not previously slowed down their metabolic rate with frequent dieting.

Most people fall somewhere between these two extremes and maintain comfortably on three meals plus the afternoon and evening snacks plus activity which usually averages four to five weekly sessions of 45-60 minutes.

There is no particular restraint on foods with the exception of keeping fat and sugar intake low. If there is a period of "overindulgence" they compensate by adding an additional 30-60 minute activity each day with strict adherence to the eating plan or they follow the "Quick Weight Loss" plan for two or three days following the "overindulgence." Otherwise, they eat a basically nutritious fare including favorite foods, and occasional desserts or other "binge" foods.

These illustrations of different approaches to maintenance should reinforce the fact that there are no two people exactly alike and you must monitor yourself, making food choices and activity changes carefully during the first weeks of maintenance. The more overweight you were at the start of the program and the more frequently you have dieted in the past will have a direct influence on the type of maintenance program you will need. Being more than 45 pounds overweight and a frequent dieter at the start may mean that you will have to do a minimum of 60 minutes of activity a day, 5 days weekly and increase activity anytime you increase food intake. Otherwise 45-60 minutes for 4-5 days weekly is the usual average and along with the eating plan works very well. These are general guidelines and it will be necessary for you to make adjustments based on your own body's response.

Make no mistake – I am not just talking about weight control. If you've been following the program even for one week, you should already be experiencing increases in energy and health benefits as well as weight loss. If you feel you don't have time for an hour of activity, then walk or bounce on the mini tramp for two 30 minute sessions each day, or walk to work in the morning or walk at lunch. Put the mini tramp in front of the T.V. in the evening and bounce through your favorite program. If weight control is a priority you will find the time just as you do for any other priority. If weight control is not a priority then your health should be. Today, even insurance companies are viewing overweight as a serious health problem and some are refusing to write policies for overweight people. They only have money to lose – you have your health to lose!

Guidelines For Your Maintenance Program

By the time you are ready to maintain your weight loss, you have already been practicing the basics of lifetime maintenance. These few suggestions will be easy to incorporate:

1. Always have 3 meals plus an afternoon snack. Other snacks are optional, but do include them if you are hungry.

2. Evening meals – the lightest of the day for a minimum of 6 days weekly.

3. Lunch – largest of the day for a minimum of 6 days weekly.

4. "Binge" day once weekly or as tolerated without weight gain. Increase activity to compensate if there is a problem or use "Quick Weight Loss" plan.

5. P/F meals or snacks – if desired, may be increased occasionally to 2 daily if tolerated.

6. Plan meals and snacks a minimum of one day in advance. This is a *must!*

7. Increase fruit intake gradually as tolerated.

8. Eat only foods you enjoy.

9. Portion sizes and amounts of food eaten should always be regulated by the rule – never stuffed, never hungry!

10. If you overindulge, always use "Quick Weight Loss" for several days or as needed.

11. Activity – 45-60 minutes three to six times weekly. Adjust as necessary.

If You Begin To Gain – Check Points

1. Adequate length and frequency of activity?

2. Exercise Heart Rate – checking and making adjustments in intensity to maintain EHR throughout activity?

3. Evening meals – too much fat or too much total food intake?

4. P/F meals and snacks – too much fat intake?

5. Fiber intake – do snacks and meals include high fiber grains and raw veggies?

6. Snacks – afternoon snack adequate? Evening snacks *light*, as they should be?

If you have checked carefully all of the above and still have a problem, it might be wise to go back to the menus provided earlier for one or two weeks or use "Quick Weight Loss" for one week to get you back "on track."

Set a goal for yourself that is reasonable. It is best if you decide on a particular size of clothes – pants, dress, belt size, etc., rather than weight. Once you're comfortably wearing that particular size, note your weight. Allow a weight fluctuation of 2-4 pounds (more for pre-menstrual days, or avoid weigh-ins at that time). Begin to increase activity and adjust eating or follow "Quick Weight Loss" plan if you gain more than 4 pounds.

To Simplify – Remember
"SAFE"

It has been my hope to simplify the "Fat To Fit" program as much as possible, without sacrificing important information you need for your success. To simplify even more, use the word "SAFE" as a memory jogger to help you focus on four of the most important scientifically based principles of the "Fat To Fit" program to increase metabolism and normalize weight.

S - Sugar intake should be kept as low as possible.

A - Activity is an absolute must. Metabolic increases produced through aerobic activity is essential.

F - Fat intake must be kept very low. Read food labels!

E - Evening eating must be light. Make sure you have a good lunch and always an afternoon snack and you will not be very hungry in the evening. If you are hungry at evening dinner, have an appetizer before you eat your meal.

Use of the above four, plus the "Quick Weight Loss," after overindulgences are the simple basics that will keep you at your desired level of weight and fitness for lifetime!

Basically the "Fat To Fit" program is a simple but scientific program that will allow you to eat the foods you enjoy, lose weight and increase your energy level without the discomfort and health risks of dieting. However, like any new behavior or skill, it must take priority for the first few weeks as you learn to work *with* your body to lose weight comfortably so that you will never go hungry or be overweight again. Giving it time and priority as you do other important skills you wish to learn, will reward you not only with permanent weight control but also energy increases and health benefits that may seem almost miraculous!

Questions – Maintenance

I absolutely love ice cream, but I know that it is high in both fat and sugar content. Could you suggest another similar food as a substitute?

You sound like my kind of person! Ice cream is *always* my "Binge Day" food! For this reason, I feel more than qualified to answer your question, and the answer is *ice milk*. Before you turn up your nose, let me tell you that today's ice milk is a great improvement over the ice milk I remember of several years ago. Some brands are much better than others, so try several brands to find one you like. I actually *prefer* ice milk over ice cream, but it is still a "Binge Day" food because of the sugar content. It is a much better choice than ice cream because the fat content is less than half!

What about maintenance while on vacation? Any special tips?

Vacations and/or extended holidays will be no problem when you *plan ahead*! If you know you'll be indulging more frequently, then plan for it and use the "Quick Weight Loss" plan one week before and again one week after. This will "rev" up the metabolism even more so that the extra calories are burned and not stored as fat. Vacations may not add the weight you fear because oftentimes you are more physically active on vacation than at your regular job. Vacations at a beach offer walking opportunities that are the very best! Fast walks on the beach have often brought people back from vacation even thinner! As far as snacks – take some with you, or purchase some from a grocery store once you arrive at your destination. Non-perishable snacks can be kept in motel rooms or even taken to the beach to munch on. Use the "Meals And Snacks - Suggestions" for ideas to help with snacks and ordering meals in restaurants.

One thing I can guarantee – if you stay active and eat sensibly with occasional "binge" foods, your energy level will be very high and you will enjoy your vacation or holidays and return home to your regular schedule totally rejuvenated! However, if you are inactive, lounge around and eat lots of sugary or fatty foods, you will feel lethargic and return home exhausted! Consider these two options when you make your plans.

Why do you suggest that evening meals should be the lightest for only 6 days weekly and not every day?

This will give you the opportunity to eat a regular-sized dinner at least once weekly if you choose. Sometimes when people eat out they would like this option, and on maintenance it should not present a problem. Others are accustomed to eating lighter evening meals and will eat a larger evening meal only on rare occasions.

Make sure you have light carbohydrates for lunch if you plan on having a larger evening meal.

Sometimes I am so tired in the evenings after work that I dread beginning my activity, but after about 15 minutes I begin feeling better and by the time I finish 50 minutes, I feel great! Why is this?

Your reaction is perfectly normal and is a good example of some of the benefits of the activity. People who jog or run call this the "runner's high" and knowing that you will experience this feeling, will help motivate you to continue to do your activity as part of your lifestyle and will also help get you started on days when you would rather not.

The reason for your increase in mental and physical energy is very simple. Activity that is aerobic triggers the release of a hormone that is a mood elevator and also an appetite depressant. This natural hormone relieves stress, depresses appetite, and acts as an "energizer." Because of this, many people taking tranquilizers find that they are able to decrease the dosage or discontinue their medication shortly after beginning a regularly scheduled aerobic activity.

How long should I continue to plan meals and snacks one day ahead?

For a lifetime! I have maintained my normal weight for ten years now, and if I don't plan and get the necessary food ready for the next day, I will invariably miss a meal or more often my afternoon snack. Schedules are hectic for everyone today and planning as well as preparing means the food will be available. Just as important, it will establish your eating plan as a priority. IF YOU FAIL TO PLAN, YOU ARE PLANNING TO FAIL!

EPILOGUE

As with any worthwhile endeavor, changing your lifestyle takes not only commitment but also time and practice. While you are "practicing" you will be losing weight, but realize also that you are certain to make mistakes. Just as the archer becomes expert by learning proper adjustments from mistakes in missing the target, you must also allow your mistakes to teach you proper adjustments. Mistakes are a necessary part of learning and the *reality* of each mistake must be accepted but not its *permanence*.

Another helpful change of perspective is to refuse to consider weight control as a "problem," but rather to consider it as a "project" on which you are working. We tend to tackle a project with great enthusiasm, determination, and the conviction that it will be done!

Now that you have the tools, it is your choice and commitment that is needed to insure your success. Within you at this moment is the possibility of success, but only you have the power to control your mind and make your choices. When you take control of your inner world of mind, external temptations will lose their power and you will not only reach your goal, but you will also gain a wonderful sense of freedom.

"Oh while I live, to be the ruler of life, not a slave, to meet life as a powerful conqueror, and nothing exterior to me shall ever take command of me." – Walt Whitman

In closing, it is my sincere belief that your weight control project will be successful, and in completing this project you will discover a most rewarding and fulfilling level of life open to you!

SOURCES

Sources of information for this book include not only books and articles but also my own formal education, seminars, symposiums, research reports, personal experiences, and data from several hundred participants in the "Fat To Fit" program. Many of the following books and articles, written by medical doctors, Ph.D.s and nutritionists, present the latest weight control research material in easy to read language and would make an excellent list of suggested reading materials.

Adibi, Siamak A. "Amino Acids and Peptide Absorption in Human Intestines: Implications for External Nutrition," In: *Amino Acids, Metabolism and Medical Applications*, John Wright, Boston, p. 255-263.

Adibi, Siamak A, Morse, Emile L. "Intestinal Transport of Dipeptides in Man: Relative Importance of Hydrolysis and Intact Absorption," *The Journal of Clinical Investigation*, Vol. 50, 1971.

Adibi, Siamak, Mercer, Donald W. "Protein Digestion in Human Intestine as Reflected in Luminal, Mucosal, and Plasma Amino Acid Concentrations After Meals," *The Journal of Clinical Investigation*, Vol. 52, July 1973.

Adibi, Siamak, and Soleimanpour, Mohammad R. "Functional Characterization of Dipeptide Transport System in Human Jejunum," *The Journal of Clinical Investigation*, Vol. 53, May 1974.

Atkins, Robert C. *Diet Revolution*. New York: David McKay Co., Inc., 1973.

Barone, Jeanine. "Immunity: A Delicate Balance," *American Health*, Dec. 1987, p. 58-61.

Bolger, James. "Fats: The Inside Story," *Family Safety & Health*, Fall 1987, p. 21-22.

Blackburn, G.L., Pavlou K. "Fad Reducing Diets: Separating Fads From Facts," *Contemporary Nutrition*, Vol. 8(7), 1983, p. 1-2.

Brody, Jane. "Nutrition Update," *New Body*, Jan. 1988, p. 19.

Brownell, Kelly. "The Yo-Yo Trap," *American Health*, May 1988, p. 78-84.

Brownell, Kelly. "The Sad Truth about Dieting," *The Washington Post*, May 27, 1987, p. E1-E9.

Butterworth, Eric. *Spiritual Economics*. Unity Village: Unity School of Christianity, 1983.

Certified Nutritionist Reference Book . Nutritionists Institute of America, Kansas City: Reg. U.S. Pat. & TM Off.

Coyle, E. F., and others. "Carbohydrate Feeding During Prolonged Strenuous Exercise Can Delay Fatigue," *American Physiological Society*, 1983.

Davis, Adelle. *Let's Eat Right To Keep Fit* . New York: Harcourt, Brace & World, Inc., 1954.

Davis, Adelle. *Let's Get Well* . New York: Harcourt, Brace & World, Inc., 1965.

Dohm, G. Lynis, and others. "Adaptation of ProteinMetabolism to Endurance Training," *Biochemistry Journal*, Vol. 164, 1977.

Dohm, G. Lynis, and others. "Changes in Tissue Protein Levels as a Result of Endurance Exercise," *Life Sciences*, Vol. 23, p. 845-850.

Ellis, Gregory. "Don't Waste Muscle: Build It!," *Muscle and Fitness*, Aug. 1983, p. 62-64.

Ernsberger, Paul. "The Death of Dieting," *American Health*, Jan./Feb. 1985, p. 29-33.

"Exercise and Osteoporosis," *Nutritionist's News* , August 1986, p. 3.

"Exercise Builds Strong Bones," University of California, *Berkeley Wellness Letter* , Jan. 1985, p. 6-7.

Gebhardt, Susan E., Matthews, Ruth H. *Nutritive Value of Foods*. Washington, D.C.: U.S. Government PrintingOffice, 1981.

Goldberg, Alfred L., Chang, Tse Wen. "Regulation and Significance of Amino Acid Metabolism in Skeletal Muscle," *Input*, 1984.

Haas, Robert. *Eat To Win*. New York: New American Library, 1983.

Hilgard, Ernest, Atkinson, Richard and Atkinson, Rita L. *Introduction To Psychology*. New York: Harcourt Brace Jovanovich, Inc., 1971.

"How RDA's Developed," *Nutritionist's News*, May 1986, p. 1.

Ivy, J. L., and others. "Endurance Improved by Ingestion of a Glucose Polymer Supplement," *Medicine and Science in Sports and Exercise*, Vol. 15, No. 6, p. 466-471.

Katahn, Martin. *Beyond Diet*. New York: Berkley Publishing Corp., 1986.

Kolata, Gina. "The Superpill Scandal," *American Health*, Jan./Feb. 1987, p. 56-57.

Kuhn, Penelope L. "Fat Or Fiction," *New Body*, June 1982, p. 21-22.

Kunur, Richard A. *Mega-Nutrition*. New York: McGraw Hill Book Co., 1981.

"Latest Findings on Obesity and Health," *Consumer's Research*, April, 1985, p. 11-15.

Lecos, Chris W. "Aspartame," *FDA Consumer*, HHS Pub. No. (FDA) 85-2205, Reprinted from Feb. 1985.

"Liquid Protein and Sudden Cardiac Deaths – An Update," *FDA Drug Bulletin*, May-June, 1978, p. 18.

Mann, John A. "Free-Form Amino Acid Mixtures Rip-Off," *Mega Health Society*, Vol. 4, 1984, Manhattan Beach, CA, 1984.

Miller, Wayne C. "The Non-Diet Diet," *Shape*, March, 1987, p. 94-96.

Mindell, Earl. *Shaping Up With Vitamins*. New York: Warner Books, Inc., 1985.

"The More Television The Fatter the Children," *Tufts University Diet & Nutrition Letter* , July 1985, p. 1.

Mathnu, Ira. "The New Nutrition," *American Health*, Sept. 1987, p. 70-74.

Mathnu, Ira. "What's Your Foodstyle?," *American Health*, Oct., 1987, p. 50-56.

Mathnu, Ira. "Our Low Energy Eats," *American Health*, Oct. 1987, p. 58-59.

McDougall, John A. and Mary A. *The McDougall Plan.* Piscataway, NJ: New Century Publishers, Inc., 1983.

"Obesity: A Growing Problem With Children," *American Institute For Cancer Research Newsletter,* Spring 1988, p. 3.

Odessey, Richard, Goldberg, Alfred L. "Oxidation of Leucine by Rat Skeletal Muscle," *American Journal of Physiology,* Vol. 223, No. 6, December 1972.

Perry, Arlette. "The Workout of the Future," *Shape,* Sept. 1987, p. 108.

"Protein – Too Much of a Good Thing?," *Running & Fitnews,* American Running and Fitness Association, May 1987, p. 3.

Remmington, Dennis, Fisher, Garth, and Parent, Edward. *How To Lower Your Fat Thermostat.* Pravo, Utah: Vitality House International, Inc., 1986.

Saltman, Paul, Gurin, Joel, and Mathnu, Ira. *The California Nutrition Book.* Toronto: Little, Brown & Co., 1987.

Shell, Ellen Ruppel. "Kids, Catfish and Cholesterol," *American Health,* Jan./Feb., 1988, p. 52-57.

Silk, D.B.A. "Amino Acid and Peptide Absorption in Man," In: *Peptide Transport and Hydrolysis* (CIBA Found. Symp. 50), 1977, p. 15-19.

Silk, D.B.A. "Absorption of Amino Acids From An Amino Acid Mixture Simulating Casein and a Tryptic Hydrolysate of Casein in Man," *Clinical Science and Molecular Medicine,* (1973) 45, p. 715-719.

Silk, D.B.A., and others. "Comparison of Oral Feeding of Peptide and Amino Acid Meals To Normal Human Subjects," *Gut*, 1979, p. 291-299.

Sours, H. "Sudden Death Associated With Very Low Calorie Weight Reduction Regimes," *American Journal Clinical Nutrition*, 34 (1981): p. 453.

Stone, Martin L. "Osteoporosis Can Be Prevented," *Health & Fitness '87*, June 22, 1987, S-29 - S-30.

Vash, Peter D. "How To Fight Fat," *Shape*, December 1987, p. 22.

Vash, Peter D. "The Second Time Around," *Shape*, April, 1988, p. 28-29.

Wade, Carlson. *Amino Acids Book.* Conn: Keats Publishing Inc., 1985.

Watt, Bernice K., Merrill, Annabel, L. "Composition of Foods," *Washington, DC: U.S. Dept. of Agriculture* , 1963.

"When The Going Gets Really Tough," University of California, *Berkeley Wellness Letter* , Jan. 1985, p. 7.

Wolfe, Robert R., and others. "Isotopic Analysis of Leucine and Urea Metabolism in Exercising Humans," *American Physiological Society*, 1982.

INDEX